European Neurology

Founded 1897 as 'Monatsschrift für Psychiatrie und Neurologie', continued 1957–1967 as 'Psychiatria et Neurologia'
Founders: C. Wernicke and Th. Ziehen. Successors: K. Bonhoeffer (1912–1938), J. Klaesi (1939–1967), E. Grünthal (1953–1967)

Proceedings of the International Congress
CHU Saint-Antoine, Paris, September 19–20, 1980

Deoxyglucose Uptake and Oxygen Consumption: a Metabolic Approach to Cerebral Function

Editors:
M. Le Poncin-Lafitte and J.R. Rapin, Paris

1 color plate, 63 figures, 24 tables, 1981

S. Karger · Basel · München · Paris · London · New York · Sydney

KARGER

Drug Dosage.

The authors and the publisher have exerted every effort to ensure that drug selection and dosage set forth in this text are in accord with current recommendations and practice at the time of publication. However, in view of ongoing research, changes in government regulations, and the constant flow of information relating to drug therapy and drug reactions, the reader is urged to check the package insert for each drug for any change in indications and dosage and for added warnings and precautions. This is particularly important when the recommended agent is a new and/or infrequently employed drug.

S. Karger AG, P.O. Box, CH–4009 Basel (Switzerland)
Printed in Switzerland by Thür AG Offsetdruck, Pratteln

Contents

Eur. Neurol. *20:* 137–145 (1981)

The Deoxyglucose Method: Theory and Practice

Louis Sokoloff

Laboratory of Cerebral Metabolism, National Institute of Mental Health, US Public Health Service, Department of Health and Human Services, Bethesda, Md., USA

Key Words. Deoxyglucose · Cerebral metabolism · Glucose utilization

Abstract. By analysis of a kinetic model of the behavior of 2-deoxyglucose and glucose in brain, an operational equation has been derived that allows the computation of the rates of glucose utilization simultaneously in all structures of the central nervous system on the basis of readily measurable variables. Localization in the central nervous system is achieved by a quantitative autoradiographic technique that provides direct visualization of the relative rates of glucose utilization in all parts of the central nervous system.

Introduction

The radioactive deoxyglucose method was developed to measure the local rates of energy metabolism simultaneously in all components of the brain in conscious laboratory animals. It was designed specifically to take advantage of the extraordinary spatial resolution made possible by quantitative autoradiography [5]. The dependence on autoradiography prescribed the use of radioactive substrates for energy metabolism, the labeled products of which could be assayed in the tissues by the autoradiographic technique. Although oxygen consumption is the most direct measure of energy metabolism, the volatility of oxygen and its metabolic products and the short physical half-life of its radioactive isotopes precluded measurement of oxidative metabolism by the autoradiographic technique. In most circumstances glucose is almost the sole substrate for cerebral oxidative metabolism, and its utilization is stoichiometrically related to oxygen consumption. Radioactive glucose is, however, not fully satisfactory because its labeled products are lost too rapidly from the cerebral tissues. The labeled analogue of glucose, 2-deoxy-*D*-[^{14}C]glucose, was, therefore, selected because its biochemical properties make it particularly appropriate to trace glucose metabolism and to measure local cerebral glucose utilization by the autoradiographic technique.

Theory

The method was derived by analysis of a model based on the biochemical properties of 2-deoxyglucose in brain (fig. 1A) [5]. 2-Deoxyglucose (DG) is transported bi-directionally between blood and brain by the same carrier that transports glucose across the blood-brain barrier. In the cerebral tissues it is phosphorylated by hexokinase to 2-deoxyglucose-6-phosphate (DG-6-P). Deoxyglucose and glucose are, therefore, competitive substrates for both blood-brain transport and hexokinase-catalyzed phosphorylation. Unlike glucose-6-phosphate, however, which is metabolized further eventually to CO_2 and water, DG-6-P cannot be converted to fructose-6-phosphate, and it is also not a substrate for glucose-6-phosphate dehydrogenase. There is relatively little glucose-6-phosphatase activity in brain and even less deoxyglucose-6-phosphatase activity. Deoxyglucose-6-phosphate, once formed, remains, therefore, essentially trapped in the cerebral tissues, at least for the duration of the experimental period.

If the interval of time is kept short enough, for example, less than 1 h, to allow the assumption of negligible loss of [^{14}C]DG-6-P from the tissues, then the quantity of [^{14}C]DG-6-P accumulated in any cerebral tissue at any given time following the introduction of [^{14}C]DG into the circulation is equal to the integral of the rate of [^{14}C]DG phosphorylation by hexokinase in that tissue during that interval of time. This integral is in turn related to the amount of glucose that has been phosphorylated over the same interval, depending on the time courses of the relative concentrations of [^{14}C]DG and glucose in the precursor pools and the Michaelis-Menten kinetic constants for hexokinase with respect to both [^{14}C]DG and glucose. With cerebral glucose consumption in a steady state, the amount of glucose phosphorylated during the interval of time equals the steady state flux of glucose through the hexokinase-catalyzed step times the duration of the interval, and the net rate of flux of glucose through this step equals the rate of glucose utilization.

These relationships can be rigorously combined into a model (fig. 1A) which can be mathematically analyzed to derive an operational equation (fig. 1B), provided that the following assumptions are made: (1) steady state for glucose (i.e., constant plasma glucose concentration and constant rate of glucose consumption) throughout the experimental period; (2) homogeneous tissue compartment within which the concentrations of [^{14}C]DG and glucose are uniform and exchange directly with the plasma; and (3) tracer concentrations of [^{14}C]DG (i.e., molecular concentrations of free [^{14}C]DG essentially equal to zero). The operational equation which defines R_i, the rate of glucose utilization per unit mass of tissue, i, in terms of measurable variables is presented in figure 1B.

The rate constants, k_1^*, k_2^*, and k_3^*, are determined in a separate group of animals by a non-linear, iterative process which provides the least squares best-fit of an equation which defines the time course of tissue ^{14}C concentration in terms of the time, the history of the plasma concentration, and the rate constants to the

Fig. 1. Theoretical basis of the radioactive deoxyglucose method for measurement of local cerebral glucose utilization [5]. **A** Diagrammatic representation of the theoretical model. C_i^* represents the total ^{12}C concentration in a single homogeneous tissue of the brain. C_P^* and C_P represent the concentrations of [^{14}C]DG and glucose in the arterial plasma, respectively; C_E^* and C_E represent their respective concentrations in the tissue pools that serve as substrates for hexokinase. C_M^* represents the concentration of [^{14}C]DG-6-P in the tissue. The constants k_1^*, k_2^*, and k_3^* represent the rate constants for carrier-mediated transport of [^{14}C]DG from plasma to tissue, for carrier-mediated transport back from tissue to plasma, and for phosphorylation by hexokinase, respectively; the constants k_1, k_2, and k_3 are the equivalent rate constants for glucose. [^{14}C]DG and glucose share and compete for the carrier that transports both between plasma and tissue and for hexokinase which phosphorylates them to their respective hexose-6-phosphates. The dashed arrow represents the possibility of glucose-6-phosphate hydrolysis by glucose-6-phosphatase activity, if any. **B** Operational equation of the radioactive deoxyglucose method and its functional anatomy. T represents the time of termination of the experimental period; λ equals the ratio of the distribution space of deoxyglucose in the tissue to that of glucose; Φ equals the fraction of glucose which once phosphorylated continues down the glycolytic pathway; and K_m^* and V_m^* and K_m and V_m represent the familiar Michaelis-Menten kinetic constants of hexokinase for deoxyglucose and glucose, respectively. The other symbols are the same as those defined in **A**.

A

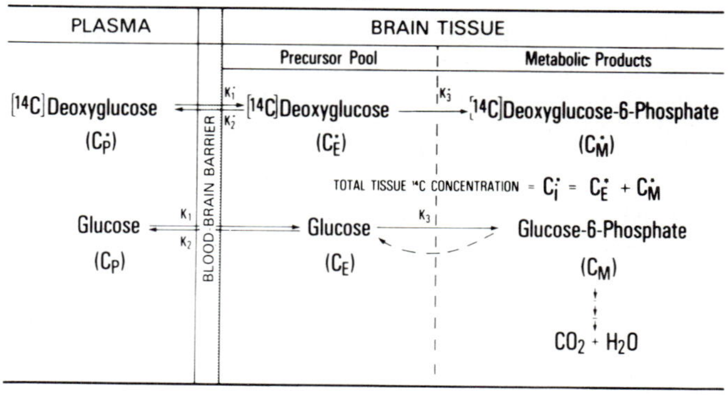

B

Functional Anatomy of the Operational Equation of the [14C] Deoxyglucose Method

General Equation for Measurement of Reaction Rates with Tracers:

$$\text{Rate of Reaction} = \frac{\text{Labeled Product Formed in Interval of Time, 0 to T}}{\left[\begin{array}{c}\text{Isotope Effect}\\ \text{Correction Factor}\end{array}\right]\left[\begin{array}{c}\text{Integrated Specific Activity}\\ \text{of Precursor}\end{array}\right]}$$

Operational Equation of [14C]Deoxyglucose Method:

$$R_i = \frac{\overbrace{\underbrace{C_i^*(T)}_{\text{Total }^{14}\text{C in Tissue at Time, T}} - \underbrace{k_1^* e^{-(k_2^*+k_3^*)T}\int_0^T C_p^* e^{(k_2^*+k_3^*)t}\,dt}_{^{14}\text{C in Precursor Remaining in Tissue at Time, T}}}^{\text{Labeled Product Formed in Interval of Time, 0 to T}}}{\underbrace{\left[\frac{\lambda\cdot V_m^*\cdot K_m}{\Phi\cdot V_m\cdot K_m^*}\right]}_{\text{Isotope Effect Correction Factor}}\underbrace{\left[\underbrace{\int_0^T \left(\frac{C_p^*}{C_p}\right)dt}_{\text{Integrated Plasma Specific Activity}} - \underbrace{e^{-(k_2^*+k_3^*)T}\int_0^T \left(\frac{C_p^*}{C_p}\right)e^{(k_2^*+k_3^*)t}\,dt}_{\text{Correction for Lag in Tissue Equilibration with Plasma}}\right]}_{\text{Integrated Precursor Specific Activity in Tissue}}}$$

experimentally determined time courses of tissue and plasma concentrations of ^{14}C [5]. The λ, Φ, and the enzyme kinetic constants are grouped together to constitute a single, lumped constant (fig. 1B). It can be shown mathematically that this lumped constant is equal to the asymptotic value of the product of the ratio of the cerebral extraction ratios of [^{14}C]DG and glucose and the ratio of the arterial blood to plasma specific activities when the arterial plasma [^{14}C]DG concentration is maintained constant [5]. The lumped constant is also determined in a separate group of animals from arterial and cerebral venous blood samples drawn during a programmed intravenous infusion which produces and maintains a constant arterial plasma [^{14}C]DG concentration [5].

Despite its complex appearance, the operational equation is really nothing more than a general statement of the standard relationship by which rates of enzyme-catalyzed reactions are determined from measurements made with radioactive tracers (fig. 1B). The numerator of the equation represents the amount of radioactive product formed in a given interval of time; it is equal to C_i^*, the combined concentrations of [^{14}C]DG and [^{14}C]DG-6-P in the tissue at time, T, measured by the quantitative autoradiographic technique, less a term that represents the free unmetabolized [^{14}C]DG still remaining in the tissue. The denominator represents the integrated specific activity of the precursor pool times a factor, the lumped constant, which is equivalent to a correction factor for an isotope effect. The term with the exponential factor in the denominator takes into account the lag in the equilibration of the tissue precursor pool with the plasma.

Procedure

The operational equation dictates the variables to be measured to determine the local rates of cerebral glucose utilization. The specific procedure employed is designed to evaluate these variables and to minimize potential errors that might occur in the actual application of the method. If the rate constants, k_1^*, k_2^*, and k_3^*, are precisely known, then the equation is generally applicable with any mode of administration of [^{14}C]DG and for a wide range of time intervals. At the present time the rate constants have been fully determined only in the conscious rat [5] (table I). Partial determination of the rate contants indicates that they are similar in the monkey [3]. These rate constants can be expected to vary with the condition of the animal, however, and for most accurate results should be redetermined for each condition studied. The structure of the operational equation suggests a more practical alternative. All the terms in the equation that contain the rate constants approach zero with increasing time if the [^{14}C]DG is so administered that the plasma [^{14}C]DG concentration also approaches zero.

From the values of the rate constants determined in normal animals and the usual time course of the clearance of [^{14}C]DG from the arterial plasma following a single intravenous pulse at zero time, it has been determined that an interval of 30–45 min after a pulse is adequate for these terms to become sufficiently small that considerable latitude in inaccuracies of the rate constants is permissible without appreciable error in the estimates of local glucose consuption [5]. An additional advantage derived from the use of a single pulse of [^{14}]DG followed by a relatively long interval before killing the animal for measurement of local tissue ^{14}C concentration is that by then most of the free [^{14}C]DG in the tissues has been either converted to [^{14}C]DG-6-P or transported back to the plasma; the optical densities in the autoradiographs then represent mainly the concentrations of [^{14}C]DG-6-P and, therefore, reflect directly the relative rates of glucose utilization in the various cerebral tissues.

The experimental procedure [5] is to inject a pulse of [^{14}C]DG intravenously at zero time and to decapitate the animal and freeze the brain at a measured time, T, 30–45 min later; in the interval timed arterial samples are taken for the measurement of plasma [^{14}C]DG and glucose concentrations. To ensure that tracer conditions are maintained, the dose of [^{14}C]DG should not exceed 2.5 μmol of deoxyglucose per kilogram of body weight. Tissue ^{14}C concentrations, C_i^*, are mesured at time, T, by quantitative autoradiography of 20 μm frozen dried sections prepared serially from the entire brain [5]. Local cerebral glucose utilization is then calculated by the operational equation.

Theoretical and Practical Considerations

Although the model and its mathematical analysis were as rigorous and comprehensive as reasonably possible, it must be recognized that models almost always represent idealized situations and cannot possibly take into account every single known, let alone unknown, property of a complex biological system. There remained, therefore, the possibility that continued experience with the [^{14}C]DG method might uncover weaknesses, limitations, or flaws serious enough to limit its usefulness or even to invalidate it. Several years have now passed since its introduction, and numerous applications of it have been made. The results of this experience generally establish the validity and worth of the method. There still remain, however, some potential problems in specialized situations, and several theoretical and practical issues need further clarification.

Rate Constants and Lumped Constant

The main potential sources of error are the rate constants and the lumped constant. The problem with them is that they are not determined in the same animals and at the same time when local cerebral glucose utilization is being measured. They are measured in separate groups of comparable animals and then used subsequently in other animals in which glucose utilization is being measured. The part played by these constants in the method is defined by their role in the operational equation of the method (fig. 1B)

Rate Constants

The rate constants, k_1^*, k_2^*, k_3^*, have thus far been fully determined for various cerebral tissues only in the normal conscious albino rat [5] (table I). Partial determination of the rate constants in the normal conscious rhesus monkey indicates that they are quite similar to those in the rat. All the rate constants vary from tissue to tissue, but the variation among gray structures and among white structures is considerably less than the differences between the two types of tissues (table I). The rate constants, k_2^* and k_3^*, appear in the equation only as their sum, and $(k_2^* + k_3^*)$ is equal to the rate constant for the turnover of the free [^{14}C]DG pool in the tissue. The half-life of the free [^{14}C]DG pool can then be calculated by dividing $(k_2^* + k_3^*)$ into the natural logarithm of 2 and has been found to average 2.4 min in gray matter and 4.5 min in white matter in the normal conscious rat (table I).

The rate constants vary not only from structure to structure but can be expected to vary with the condition. For example, k_1^* and k_2^* are influenced by both blood flow and transport of [^{14}C]DG across the blood-brain barrier, and because of the competition for the transport carrier, the glucose concentrations in the plasma and tissue affect the transport of [^{14}C]DG and, therefore, also k_1^* and k_2^*. The constant, k_3^*, is related to phosphorylation of [^{14}C]DG and will certainly change when glucose utilization is altered. To minimize potential errors due to inaccuracies in the values of the rate constants used, it was decided to sacrifice time resolution for accuracy. If the [^{14}C]DG is given as an intravenous pulse and sufficient time is allowed for the plasma to be cleared of the tracer, then the influence of the rate constants, and the functions that they represent, on the final result diminishes with increasing time until ultimately it becomes zero. This relationship is implicit in the structure of the operational equation (fig. 1B); as C_P^* approaches zero, then the terms containing the rate constants also approach zero with increasing time. The significance of this relationship is graphically illustrated in figure 2. From typical arterial plasma [^{14}C]DG and glucose concentration curves obtained in a normal conscious rat, the portion of the denominator of the operational equation underlined by the heavy bar

Table I. Values of rate constants in the normal conscious albino rat

	Rate constants, min^{-1}						Distribution volume ml/g	Half-life of precursor pool min
	k_1^*		k_2^*		k_3^*		$k_1^*/(k_2^*+k_3^*)$	$\log_e 2/(k_2^*+k_3^*)$
Gray matter								
Visual cortex	0.189	0.048	0.279	0.176	0.063	0.040	0.553	2.03
Auditory cortex	0.226	0.068	0.241	0.198	0.067	0.057	0.734	2.25
Parietal cortex	0.194	0.051	0.257	0.175	0.062	0.045	0.608	2.17
Sensorimotor cortex	0.193	0.037	0.208	0.112	0.049	0.035	0.751	2.70
Thalamus	0.188	0.045	0.218	0.144	0.053	0.043	0.694	2.56
Medial geniculate body	0.219	0.055	0.259	0.164	0.055	0.040	0.697	2.21
Lateral geniculate body	0.172	0.038	0.220	0.134	0.055	0.040	0.625	2.52
Hypothalamus	0.158	0.032	0.226	0.119	0.043	0.032	0.587	2.58
Hippocampus	0.169	0.043	0.260	0.166	0.056	0.040	0.535	2.19
Amygdala	0.149	0.028	0.235	0.109	0.032	0.026	0.558	2.60
Caudate-putamen	0.176	0.041	0.200	0.140	0.061	0.050	0.674	2.66
Superior colliculus	0.198	0.054	0.240	0.166	0.046	0.042	0.692	2.42
Pontine gray matter	0.170	0.040	0.246	0.142	0.037	0.033	0.601	2.45
Cerebellar cortex	0.225	0.066	0.392	0.229	0.059	0.031	0.499	1.54
Cerebellar nucleus	0.207	0.042	0.194	0.111	0.038	0.035	0.892	2.99
Mean	0.189		0.245		0.052		0.647	2.39
± SEM	0.012		0.040		0.010		0.073	0.40
White matter								
Corpus callosum	0.085	0.015	0.135	0.075	0.019	0.033	0.552	4.50
Genu of corpus callosum	0.076	0.013	0.131	0.075	0.019	0.034	0.507	4.62
Internal capsule	0.077	0.015	0.134	0.085	0.023	0.039	0.490	4.41
Mean	0.079		0.133		0.020		0.516	4.51
± SEM	0.008		0.046		0.020		0.171	0.90

From *Sokoloff* et al. [5].

was computed with a wide range of values for $(k_2^* + k_3^*)$ as a function of time. The values for $(k_2^* + k_3^*)$ are presented as their equivalent half-lives calculated as described above. The values of $(k_2^* + k_3^*)$ vary from infinite (i.e., $T_{1/2} = 0$ min) to 0.14 per min (i.e., $T_{1/2} = 5$ min) and more than cover the range of values to be expected under physiological conditions. The portion of the equation underlined and computed represents the integral of the precursor pool specific activity in the tissue. The curves represent the time course of this function, one each for every value of $(k_2^* + k_3^*)$ examined. It can be seen that these curves are widely different at early times but converge with increasing time until at 45 min the differences over the entire range of $(k_2^* + k_3^*)$ equal only a small fraction of the value of the

OPERATIONAL EQUATION:

$$R_i = \frac{C_i^*(T) - k_1^* e^{-(k_2^* + k_3^*)T} \int_0^T C_p^* e^{(k_2^* + k_3^*)t}\, dt}{\left(\frac{\lambda V_m^* K_m}{\Phi V_m K_m^*}\right)\left[\underline{\int_0^T (C_p^*/C_p)\, dt - e^{-(k_2^* + k_3^*)T} \int_0^T (C_p^*/C_p)\, e^{(k_2^* + k_3^*)t}\, dt}\right]}$$

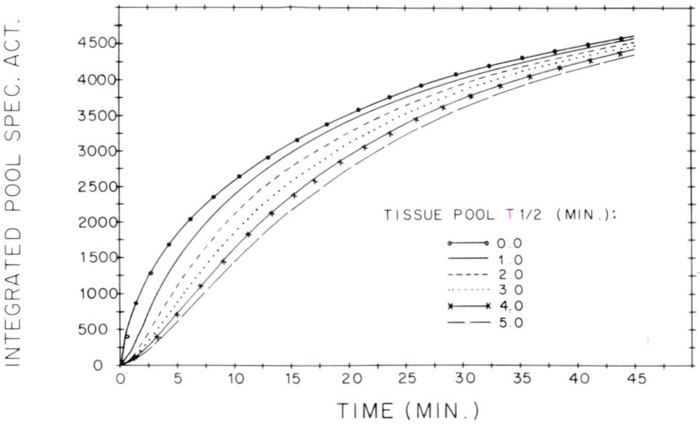

Fig. 2. Influence of time and rate constants, (k_2^* + k_3^*), on the integrated precursor pool specific activity following a pulse of [14C]DG at zero time. The portion of the equation that is underlined corresponds to the integrated pool specific activity; it was computed as a function of time with different values of (k_2^* + k_3^*), as indicated by their equivalent half-lives, calculated according to $T_{1/2} = 0.693/(k_2^* + k_3^*)$ (see text).

integral. These curves demonstrate that at short times enormous errors can occur if the values of the rate constants are not precisely known, but only negligible errors occur at 45 min, even over a wide range of rate constants of several fold. In fact, it was precisely for this reason that [^{14}C]DG rather than [^{14}C]glucose was selected as the tracer for glucose metabolism. The relationships are similar for glucose. Because the products of [^{14}C]glucose metabolism are so rapidly lost from the tissues, it is necessary to limit the experimental period to short times when enormous errors can occur if the rate constants are not precisely known. [^{14}C]DG permits the prolongation of the experimental period to times when inaccuracies in rate constants have little effect on the final result.

It should be noted, however, that in pathological conditions, such as severe ischemia or hyperglycemia, the rate constants may fall far beyond the range examined in figure 2. We have evidence, for example, that this occurs with arterial plasma glucose concentrations above 300 mg%. In such abnormal conditions it may be necessary to redetermine the rate constants for the particular condition under study.

Lumped Constant

The lumped constant is composed of six separate constants. One of these, Φ, is a measure of the steady-state hydrolysis of glucose-

Table II. Values of the lumped constant in the albino rat, rhesus monkey, cat and dog

Animal	Number of animals	Mean ± SD	SEM
Albino rat			
Conscious	15	0.464 ± 0.099[1]	0.026
Anesthetized	9	0.512 ± 0.118[1]	0.039
Conscious (5% CO_2)	2	0.463 ± 0.122[1]	0.086
Combined	26	0.481 ± 0.119	0.023
Rhesus monkey			
Conscious	7	0.344 ± 0.095	0.036
Cat			
Anesthetized	6	0.411 ± 0.013	0.005
Dog (Beagle puppy)			
Conscious	7	0.558 ± 0.082	0.031

[1] No statistically significant difference between normal conscious and anesthetized rats ($0.3 < p < 0.4$) and conscious rats breathing 5% CO_2 ($p > 0.9$).

Note: The values were obtained as follows: rat [5]; monkey [3]; cat (*Miyaoka, Magnes, Kennedy, Shinohara, Sokoloff,* unpublished data); dog [1].

6-phosphate to free glucose and phosphate. Because in normal brain tissue there is little such phosphohydrolase activity [2], Φ is normally approximately equal to unity. The other components are arranged in three ratios: λ, which is the ratio of distribution spaces in the tissue for deoxyglucose and glucose; V^*_m/V_m; and K_m/K^*_m. Although each individual constant may vary from structure to structure and condition to condition, it is likely that the ratios tend to remain the same under normal conditions. For reasons described in detail previously [5], it is reasonable to believe that the lumped constant is the same throughout the brain and is characteristic of the species of animal, but only in normal tissue. Although reasonable, it is not certain, and there are theoretical possibilities that it may not be so. Empirical experience thus far indicates that it is. The greatest experience has been accumulated in the albino rat. In this species the lumped constant for the brain as a whole has been determined under a variety of conditions [5]. In the normal conscious rat local cerebral glucose utilization, determined by the [^{14}C]DG method with the single value of the lumped constant for the brain as a whole, correlates almost perfectly ($r = 0.96$) with local cerebral blood flow, measured by the [^{14}C]iodoantipyrine method, an entirely independent method [4]. It is generally recognized that local blood flow is adjusted to local metabolic rate, but if the single value of the lumped constant did not apply to the individual structures studied, then errors in local glucose utilization would occur that might be expected to obscure the correlation. Also, the lumped constant has been directly determined in the albino rat in the normal conscious state, under barbiturate anesthesia, and during the inhalation of 5% CO_2; no significant differences were observed (table II). The lumped constant does vary with the species of animal. It has now also been determined in the Rhesus monkey [3], cat [*Miyaoka, Magnes, Kennedy, Shinohara, Sokoloff,* unpublished data], and Beagle puppy [1], and each species has a different value (table II). The values for local rates of glucose utilization determined with these lumped constants in these species are very close to what might be expected from measurement of energy metabolism in the brain as a whole by other methods.

References

1 Duffy, T.E.; Cavazzuti, M.; Gregoire, N.M.; Cruz, N.F.; Kennedy, C.; Sokoloff, L.: Regional cerebral glucose metabolism in newborn beagle dogs. Trans. Am. Soc. Neurochem. *10:* 171 (1979).
2 Hers, H.G.: Le métabolisme du fructose, p. 102 (Editions Arscia, Bruxelles 1957).
3 Kennedy, C.; Sakurada, O.; Shinohara, M.; Jehle, J.; Sokoloff, L.: Local cerebral glucose utilization in the normal conscious Macaque monkey. Ann. Neurol. *4:* 293–301 (1978).
4 Sokoloff, L.: Local cerebral energy metabolism: its relationships to local functional activity and blood flow; in Cerebral vascular smooth muscle and its control. Ciba Fdn Symp. 56 (new series), pp. 171–191 (Elsevier/Excerpta Medica/North-Holland, Amsterdam 1978).
5 Sokoloff, L.; Reivich, M.; Kennedy, C.; Des Rosiers, M.H.; Patlak, C.S.; Pettigrew, K.D.; Sakurada, O.; Shinohara, M.: The [^{14}C]deoxyglucose method for the measurement of local cerebral glucose utilization: theory, procedure, and normal values in the conscious and anesthetized albino rat. J. Neurochem. *28:* 897–916 (1977).

Louis Sokoloff, MD, Laboratory of Cerebral Metabolism, National Institute of Mental Health, US Public Health Service, Department of Health and Human Services, Bethesda, MD 20205 (USA)

Eur. Neurol. *20:* 146–151 (1981)

Deoxyglucose Uptake in Pathological Conditions

J.R. Rapin, A. Lageron, M. Le Poncin-Lafitte
Neurophysiologie cérébrovasculaire, CHU St-Antoine, Paris, France

Key Words. Deoxyglucose uptake · Hypoxia · Stricture · Ischemia

Abstract. In case of quick physiological variations or in pathological conditions, it is impossible to measure the deoxyglucose consumption by means of the deoxyglucose technique and we propose a method for the study of the deoxyglucose uptake by the cerebral tissue. It is simultaneously measured with the blood flow, 3 min following the intravenous administration of deoxyglucose (2-deoxyglucose-^{14}C). Hypercapnia induces an increase in the flow but does not modify the deoxyglucose uptake and moderate hypoxia results in a decrease in the deoxyglucose uptake without modifying the flow. In pathological conditions such as ischemia or stricture, the blood flow and deoxyglucose uptake variations are not parallel. These results show that the 2-deoxyglucose uptake does not follow the blood flow and that it depends on the cell activity. It is therefore possible to use this method when the consumption studies cannot be implemented.

Introduction

Deoxyglucose is trapped by the cerebral tissue in the same conditions as glucose and both substances compete to be phosphorylated by hexokinase. Deoxyglucose-6-phosphate cannot be metabolized and its accumulation allows to measure the glucose uptake according to a method of quantitative autoradiography [7]. This determination however must be performed in a steady state and requires a time interval of about 30 or 45 min after the administration of labelled deoxyglucose. The time interval is incompatible with quick physiological variations such as paradoxical sleep, learning and memorization processes. Besides, in pathological cases, the steady state conditions are no longer respected and it is no longer possible to study the glucose consumption.

In such cases, it seemed interesting to us to apply a method for determining the deoxyglucose uptake. In fact, it may be assumed that the cell activity controlling the activity of hexokinase also controls the intake of sugar at the level of its uptake.

Deoxyglucose was prefered to glucose because it is not degraded and it is easy to study the plasmatic pharmacokinetics. Moreover, since the steady state conditions are no longer respected, it is necessary to simultaneously determine the deoxyglucose uptake and the local blood flow.

Method

The animals were male Sprague-Dawley rats. A catheter was surgically introduced into the jugular vein and another one into the caudal artery. 48 h later, deoxyglucose-^{14}C (100 μCi/kg) was intravenously administered, and 2 min 30 s later, iodoantipyrine-^{125}I (100 μCi/kg). Exactly 30 s after the latter administration, the animals were decapitated. During these 3 min, arterial blood was sampled in order to determine the kinetics of deoxyglucose and the average cardiac output. Hematocrit was determined as well as the glucose level, measured according to the method of glucose oxidase.

The brain was rapidly removed and divided into the hypothalamus, the cerebellum, the midbrain, the striatum, the hippocampus and the cortex on a cooled plate. The deoxyglucose-^{14}C radioactivity in these various structures was measured by means of liquid scintillation; the window was adjusted so as to avoid contamination by iodine-125, the radioactivity of which was determined in a gamma spectrometer. The deoxyglucose uptake was expressed as a percentage of the injected radioactivity and the local flows in ml/min/100 g.

Pathological Models

Environmental Changes. Groups of 6 rats were exposed to specific environmental conditions. One group was placed in a closed space ventilated with a mixture of 14% oxygen and 86% nitrogen for 30 min. Another group was placed in a closed space with 5% CO_2 for 30 min.

Model for Anoxia or Ischemia. A 1-min stricture was performed in one group, thus completely stopping the blood circulation. The deoxyglucose uptake and the blood flow were studied during the recirculation stage, 3 and 6 min after the end of the stricture. In the other group, a quantitative ischemia was obtained by the injection of 2,000 microspheres into the internal carotid via the external carotid. 15 min, 1, 2, 3, 4, 6 and 24 h later the deoxyglucose uptake and the blood flow were determined according to the above-described method.

Results

Effects of Hypoxia and CO_2 on Deoxyglucose Uptake and Blood Flow (table I)

Moderate normobaric hypoxia results in a decrease in the deoxyglucose uptake without causing a flow variation in the total brain. Similar results were found at the level of the various structures. Hypercapnia entails a significant decrease in the cerebral blood flow with no noteworthy change in the deoxyglucose uptake. However, at the level of the bulb, there is an increase both in the blood flow and in the deoxyglucose uptake. The variations observed at the level of the other structures are of the same order than those reported for the total brain.

Table I. Effects of normobaric hypoxia (oxygen 14%) and CO^2 (5%) on the deoxyglucose uptake and the blood flow in whole brain

	Blood flow ml/min/100 g	Deoxyglucose uptake, %
Control	48 ± 2	2.3 ± 0.1
Hypoxia	48 ± 4	1.6 ± 0.1**
Hypercapnia	62 ± 3**	2.4 ± 0.2

Mean ± SEM (n = 6).
** $p \leq 0.01$.

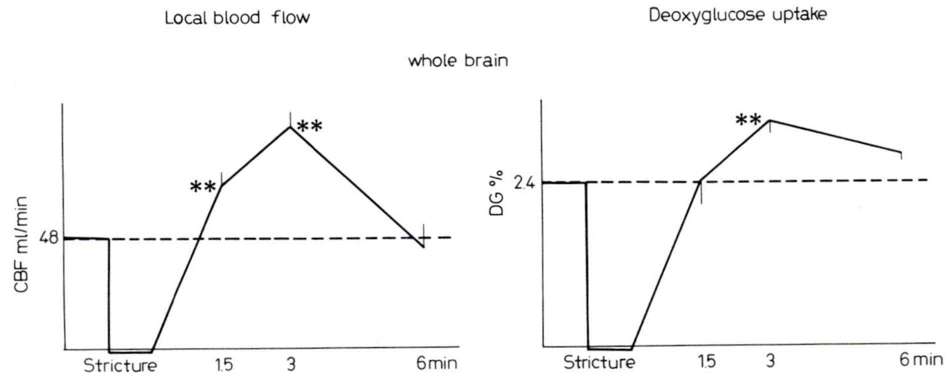

Fig. 1. Effect of stricture (1 min) on the deoxyglucose uptake (DG) and the cerebral blood flow (CBF) during the recirculation period in whole brain. Each point is the mean ± SEM of 6 determinations. $^{**}p \leqslant 0.01$.

Effects of Stricture on Deoxyglucose Uptake and Cerebral Blood Flow

After a 1-min stricture, an increase in the blood flow was observed for a few minutes during recirculation and this was associated to an increase in the deoxyglucose uptake. This result was observed in the whole brain (fig. 1) and also in the various structures, particularly in the hypothalamus and striatum (fig. 2).

Effect of Quantitative Embolization on Deoxyglucose Uptake and Cerebral Blood Flow

Labelled microspheres allow to quantify the embolization and to determine their localization [1, 4]. After the embolization, the cerebral blood flow decreases by about 50% in the embolized side whereas it remains normal or near to its normal value in the nonembolized side. The decrease remains very important in the 24 h following the embolization. The evolution of the deoxyglucose uptake is different. It decreases in the 1st hour and on the contrary, an increase was observed as soon as the 4th or 5th hour (fig. 3).

Discussion

Deoxyglucose uptake occurs in the same conditions as glucose and is rapidly phosphorylated in the cells. The radioactivity measured at the level of the brain in the first minutes after the administration of the substances corresponds only to nonphosphorylated deoxyglucose [6]. Consequently, choosing a time interval of 3 min after the administration, we studied the deoxyglucose uptake

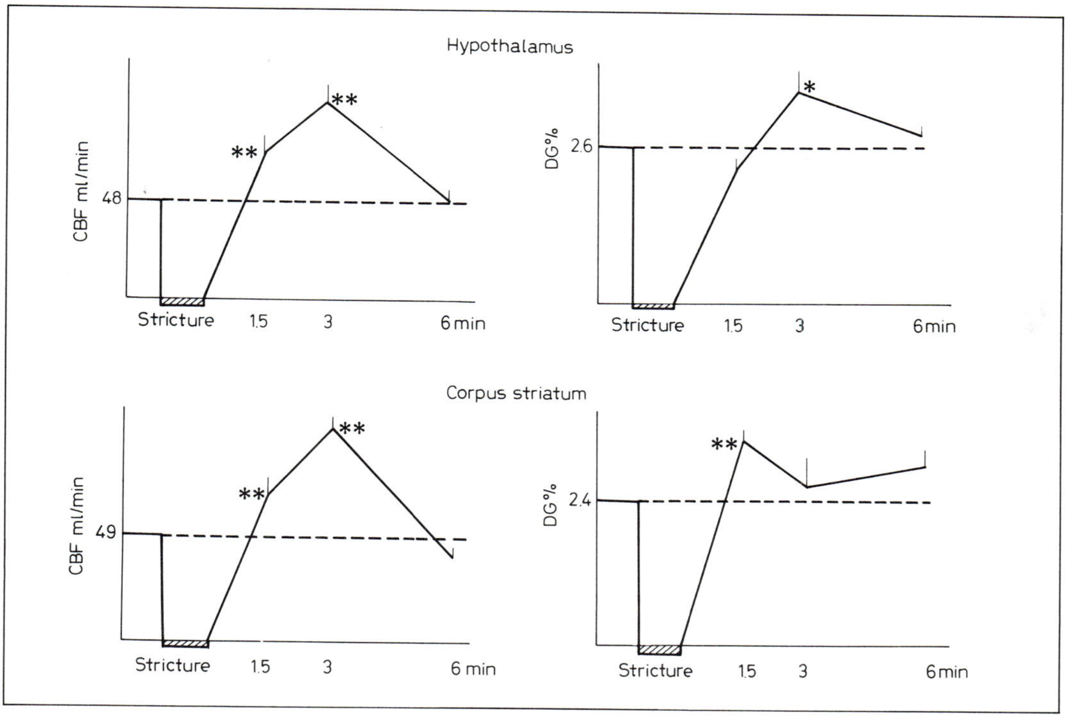

2

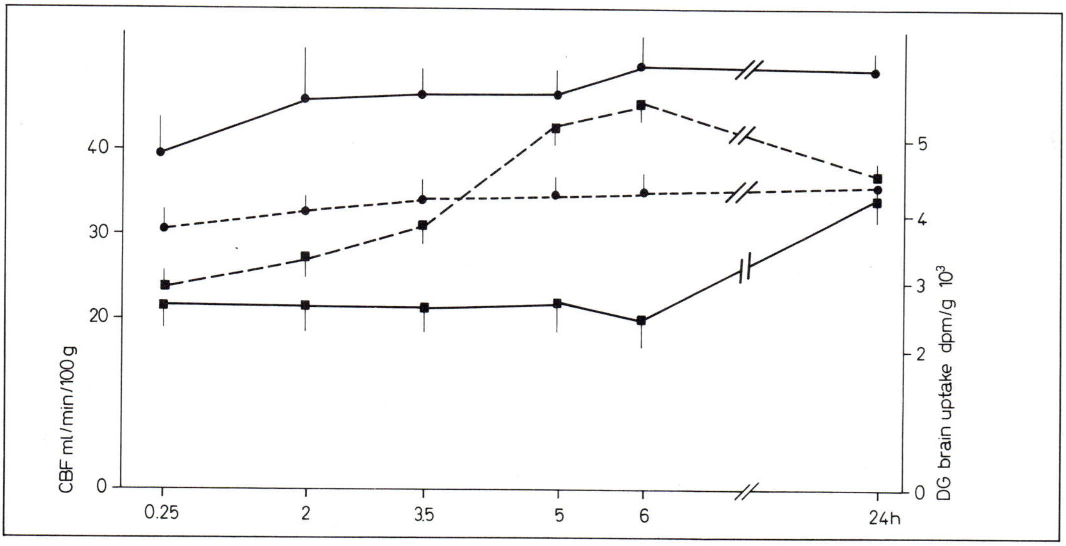

3

Fig. 2. Effect of stricture on the deoxyglucose uptake and the local blood flow during the recirculation period in hypothalamus and corpus striatum.

Fig. 3. Effect of quantitative embolization on the deoxyglucose uptake and the cerebral blood flow in whole brain. ● = Control side, —— = CBF, --- = DG uptake; ■ = embolized side, —— = CBF, --- = DG uptake.

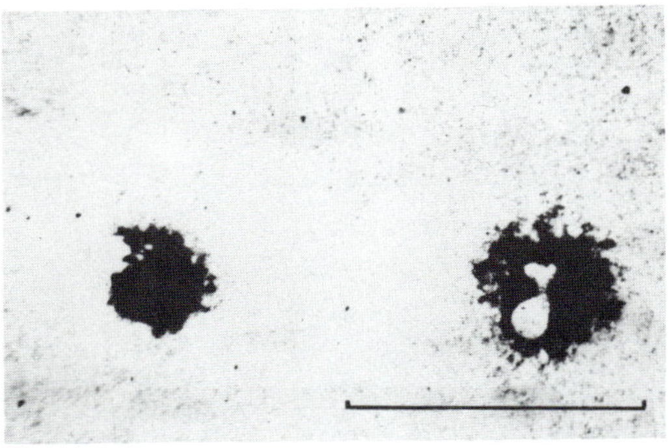

Fig. 4. Autohistoradiography obtained 3 min after the administration of labelled deoxyglucose. └─┘ = 20 µm.

at the level of the endothelium and glial cells, as is shown in figure 4. It shows the autohistoradiography obtained 3 min after administration of deoxyglucose and radioactivity was only found around the lumen of the capillary. Although the uptake in no way represents a glucose consumption, it may be related to the consumption. In fact, the nerve activity controls phosphorylations and it may be assumed that it also controls the glucose intake. In these conditions, an uptake increase would correspond to any hyperactivity, and contrarily, in the case of hypoactivity, there would be a decrease in the uptake. However, glucose uptake depends on the blood flow and the transport systems and it was logical to think that both phenomena evolved in the same direction.

Our results demonstrate that the deoxyglucose uptake is independent on the blood flow and only depends on the nerve activity. In fact, the increase in the flow by CO_2 does not change the deoxyglucose uptake. Besides, low level hypoxia which simultaneously decreases the nerve activity and the deoxyglucose uptake does not induce any variation in the cerebral blood flow; hypobaric hypoxia would have resulted in an increase in the flow and in the deoxyglucose uptake [3]. Eventually, in case of ischemia, the flow is quite reduced whereas the deoxyglucose uptake is unimportant first and becomes more important 4–5 h after ischemia [5]. The parallel evolution of the flow and deoxyglucose after strangulation demonstrates the needs of the cell for glucose in the post-anoxic time interval [2]. It can be noticed that as soon as the 6th min, the deoxyglucose uptake and flow returned to their normal values, hence the absence of variation in the uptake observed 45 min later.

On the whole, these results show that there are differences between the cerebral blood flow and the deoxyglucose uptake on one side (it is therefore necessary to simultaneously measure both parameters), and that the deoxyglucose uptake may be modified as a function of the nerve activity on the other side. These findings show the interest presented by the method of deoxyglucose uptake in the short-lasting physiological responses and in pathological processes.

References

1 Bralet, A.M.; Rochette, L.; Rapin, J.R.; Bralet, J.: Localisation et effets à court terme d'une embolisation cérébrale réalisée chez le rat par injection intracarotidienne de microsphères. J. Pharmacol., Paris *8:* 241 (1977).

2 Le Poncin-Lafitte, M.; Boismare, F.; Rapin, J.R.: Effects of strangulation on deoxyglucose uptake and blood flow in the rat brain areas. Acta neurol. scand. *60:* suppl. 72, pp. 334–335 (1979).

3 Rapin, J.R.; Servin, A.; Bralet, J.: The effect of hypobaric hypoxia on cerebral uptake of ^{3}H-deoxyglucose and norepinephrine turnover rate in rats. Acta neurol. scand. *56:* suppl. 64, pp. 358–359 (1977).

4 Rapin, J.R.; Le Poncin-Lafitte, M.; Pesquies, P.C.; Lageron, A.: Troubles expérimentaux de la microcirculation cérébrale; in Pathogénie des maladies cérébrovasculaires. Symp. int., Paris, pp. 183–189 (Ipsen, Paris 1978).
5 Rapin, J.R.; Le Poncin-Lafitte, M.: Lack of correlation between cerebral blood flow and uptake of deoxyglucose after acute quantitative ischemia; in Bes, Geraud, Circulation cérébrale, pp. 89–91 (Fournié, Toulouse 1979).
6 Rapin, J.R.; Duterte, D.; Le Poncin-Lafitte, M.: Modèles d'étude des désordres cérébrovasculaires à l'aide de déoxyglucose-^{3}H. Radioakt. Isotope Klin. Forsch. *14:* 269–276 (1980).
7 Sokoloff, L.; Reivich, M.; Kennedy, C.; Des Rosiers, H.; Patlak, C.S.; Pettigrew, K.D.; Sakurada, O.; Shinohara, M.: The ^{14}C-deoxyglucose method for the measurement of local cerebral glucose utilization: theory, procedure and normal values in the conscious and anesthetized albino rat. J. Neurochem. *28:* 897–916 (1977).

J.R. Rapin, Cerebrovascular Neurophysiology Department, CHU St-Antoine,
27, rue de Chaligny, F–75012 Paris (France)

Eur. Neurol. *20:* 152–156 (1981)

The Deoxyglucose Method for Insects: towards Electron Microscopical Resolution

E. Buchner, S. Buchner

Max-Planck-Institut für biologische Kybernetik, Tübingen, BRD

Key Words. 2-Deoxy-*D*-glucose · Tritium · Autoradiography · Electron microscopical resolution · Insects · *Drosophila*

Abstract. The problems of extending the deoxyglucose method for insects to electron microscopical resolution are discussed. It is calculated that several curies of ^{3}H-deoxyglucose per kilogram body weight may be needed for identification of activity in ultra-thin sections. Oral application may be superior to injection. Incorporation of experimental and control stimulus in the same animal seems appropriate. Freeze-drying may turn out to be the best method of preparing the tissue for plastic embedding. The problem of cutting on a water surface is discussed. It is demonstrated that freeze-drying of *Drosophila* results in structural preservation sufficient for cell identification in the cervical connective. Autoradiography of ultra-thin sections has not yet been carried out.

The visual system of insects, notably flies, has become one of the model systems in neurobiology. Visually guided flight performance reflects a high level of visual information processing in this system which, on the other hand, appears less complex than the visual system of vertebrates. Considerable effort has been devoted to analyzing this system at four levels: (i) black-box analysis by behavioral experiments [9, 10], (ii) functional dissection by genetic techniques [5], (iii) single-cell analysis by electrophysiology [6] and (iv) structural analysis [12]. A major limitation, however, is represented by the fact that only a fraction of a percent of the cells in this system are large enough to be impaled by microelectrodes for intracellular recording and identification by dye injection [7]. Recently it has been demonstrated that the visual system of the fruitfly *Drosophila melanogaster* is well suited for analysis by the radioactive deoxyglucose method at a new level which lies between input-output experiments and single-cell recordings [2, 3]. In this report some of the problems are discussed that are encountered as one tries to reach single-cell resolution by the deoxyglucose method in combination with electron microscopical autoradiography.

Dosage of ^{3}H-Deoxyglucose

One of the problems of the deoxyglucose method is that *all* cells take up and phosphorylate deoxyglucose. Increase in radioactivity of a given brain region due to nervous activity usually amounted to not more than a factor of about 2–3 compared to the resting state [8, 11]. If one makes the assumption that a similar ratio of about 2 may also be expected to be found between individual active and inactive cells, one can calculate the dosage required to give a significant difference in the number of silver grains n over an active (n_1) and an inactive (n_2) cell profile of, e.g. 1 μm^2 cross-section in an autoradiograph of an ultra-thin section of 0.1 μm thickness. As the standard deviation of n is given by $\sqrt{n}$ one finds for a difference of 3 SD or a probability of accidental occurrence of $p < 0.0027$:

$$n_1 - n_2 = 2n - n = n \overset{!}{=} 3 \cdot \sqrt{(\sqrt{2n})^2 + (\sqrt{n})^2} = 3\sqrt{3} \cdot \sqrt{n}$$

or n = 27. Assuming an autoradiographic efficiency of 0.17 [1] one needs about 160 disintegrations per 0.1 μm^3 of brain tissue, or about 20 Ci/kg brain weight if homogeneous distribution throughout the brain is supposed for the labeled deoxyglucose. This is about 10^4-fold higher than has been used in vertebrates so far; it is, however, of the same order as applied to insects [2].

Application of Deoxyglucose

Stimulus-specific labeling in insects so far has been achieved only when the radioactive sugar was *fed* to the animal. One experiment in which 10 μCi of ^{3}H-deoxyglucose was injected into the hemocele of *Drosophila* (weight 1 mg) failed to provide sufficient concentration of radioactive material in the brain. Rather, most of the radioactivity was located in fuel storage compartments, i.e. the fat body. Incubation time between injection and freeze-fixation was 6 h as in feeding experiments. It is known from metabolic measurements on larger flies [13] that injected glucose is removed from the hemolymph at a 1/e rate of about 15 min. This is very short compared to the 6-hour incubation period. The successful feeding experiments therefore suggest that 'oral' application in insects may raise the concentration of deoxyglucose in the hemolymph above normal glucose levels for a period of several hours.

Stimulation

The deoxyglucose method for insects at present is only qualitatively reproducible. For quantitative comparison of activity in stimulated and unstimulated cells it will be useful to incorporate experimental and control situations in the same preparation. In this context the retinotopic organization of the optic ganglia may prove valuable as it allows one to compare the effects of various visual stimuli which may be simultaneously presented to different eye regions in one and the same animal.

Preparation

Our present procedure includes freezing in melting nitrogen, freeze-drying at −70 °C, fixation in OsO_4 vapor, dry cutting of semithin sections (2–3 μm thickness) and dry autoradiography on 'stripping film' (AR-10,

Kodak). Embedding in Epon represents the only liquid phase the tissue is exposed to after it had been frozen. Diffusion of radioactive material into spaces devoid of organic material (e.g. airsacks) is not observed. Thus it can be assumed that the autoradiographs reflect the true distribution of label at the time of freezing. Alternative procedures such as fixation in aqueous solutions and dehydration at room temperature [4] apparently do not preserve stimulus-induced distribution of label in *Drosophila* [2]. Preliminary experiments using freeze *substitution* in order to improve ultrastructural preservation of the tissue indicate that even anhydrous acetone at −70 °C may cause some diffusion of label during the process of ice dissolution [*Nicod and Buchner,* in preparation].

A final problem remains to be discussed: As there is no routine technique for cutting ultra-thin sections on a dry knife, the effect of water on the embedded tissue has to be investigated. Figure 1a shows the autoradiograph of a section to which, prior to exposure, a drop of water had been applied. The boundaries of the water droplet are clearly marked by silver grains indicating that some radioactive material has been dissolved in the water penetrating the Epon. However, enlargement of this section (fig. 1b) and comparison with the adjacent section which had not been exposed to water (fig. 1c) shows that most of the radioactive material is retained in situ. In

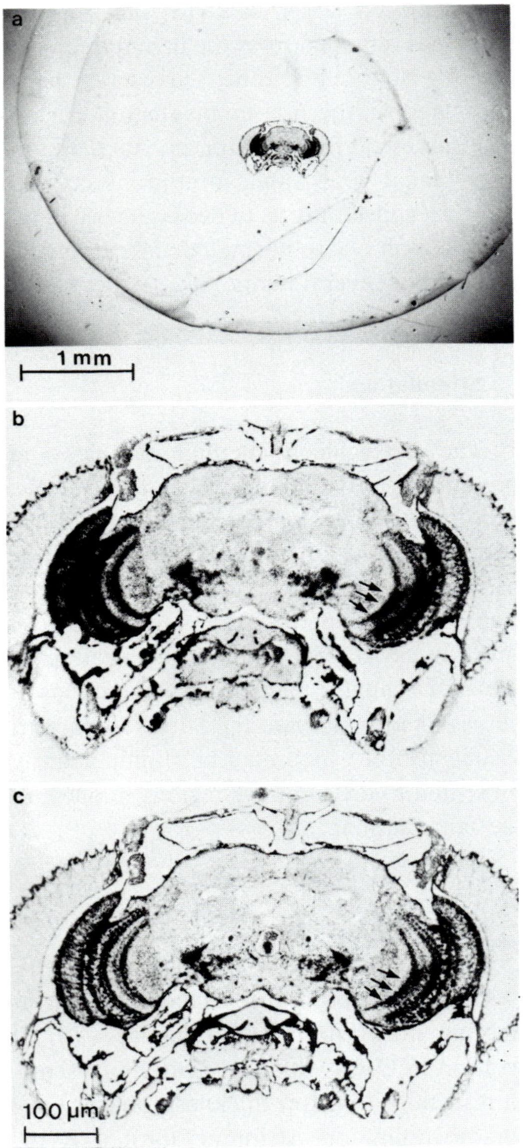

Fig. 1. Demonstration of the effect of water applied to a 3-µm thick Epon section of a *Drosophila* head. The ring of silver grains surrounding the section in the autoradiograph in **a** marks the boundary of the water droplet and indicates that some radioactive material is displaced by the water. However, comparison of this autoradiograph (enlarged in **b**) with one of the adjacent dry section (**c**) shows that even fine details of the distribution of label are preserved, in particular those of the stimulus-induced activity in the right optic ganglion (arrows). (The corresponding region of the right eye was stimulated by a moving pattern [2].)

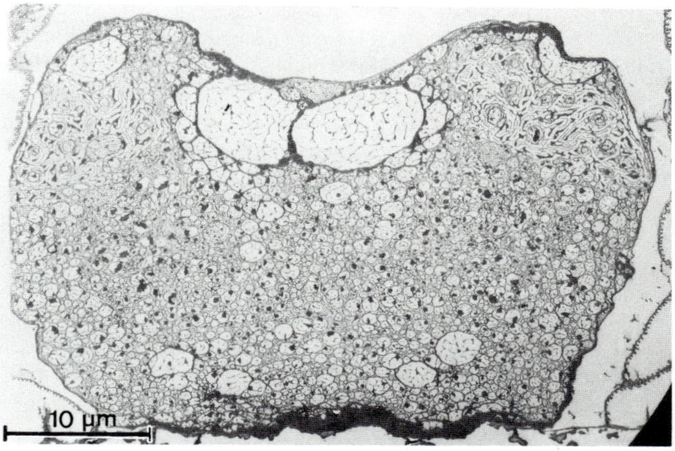

Fig. 2. Electron micrograph of the cervical connective of *Drosophila* illustrating structural preservation obtained by the present procedure. The preparation has been frozen, freeze-dried, fixed in OsO_4 vapor and embedded in Epon. Preservation of cytoplasmic membranes appears to be sufficient for cell identification. Dark patches are poorly preserved mitochondria.

particular, stimulus-induced activity (arrows) is very similar in both autoradiographs. Thus cutting on a water surface may be permissible.

Conclusion

It appears that metabolic functional mapping at the level of electron microscopical resolution should be possible if structural preservation as obtained by the freeze-drying procedure is sufficient for individual cell profiles to be identified. That this is the case with *Drosophila* is demonstrated by figure 2 which shows an electron micrograph of the cervical connective of a freeze-dried fruitfly. The cytoplasmic membranes of the nerve axons seem to be largely intact whereas subcellular structure is poorly preserved. The dark intracellular patches are mitochondria.

The non-trivial problem of adapting the technique of electron microscopical autoradiography [1] to the present preparation remains to be solved.

References

1 Bouteille, M.: The 'LIGOP' method for routine ultrastructural autoradiography. J. Microsc. Biol. cell. *27:* 121–127 (1976).

2 Buchner, E.; Buchner, S.: Mapping stimulus-induced nervous activity in small brains by ^{3}H-2-deoxy-*D*-glucose. Cell Tiss. Res. (in press, 1980).

3 Buchner, E.; Buchner, S.; Hengstenberg, R.: 2-Deoxy-*D*-glucose maps movement-specific nervous activity in the second visual ganglion of *Drosophila.* Science *205:* 687–688 (1979).

4 Des Rosiers, M.H.; Descarries, L.: Adaptation de la méthode au désoxyglucose à l'échelle cellulaire: préparation histologique du système nerveux central en vue de la radio-autographie à haute résolution. C.r. hebd. Séanc. Acad. Sci., Paris, Ser. D *287:* 153–156 (1978).

5 Hall, J.C.; Greenspan, R.J.: Genetic analysis of *Drosophila* neurobiology. A. Rev. Genet. *13:* 127–195 (1979).

6 Hausen, K.: Signal processing in the insect eye; in Stent, Function and formation of neural systems, pp. 81–110 (Dahlem Konferenzen, Berlin 1977).

7 Hengstenberg, R.: Spike responses of 'non-spiking' visual interneurones. Nature, Lond. *270:* 338–340 (1977).

8 Plum, F.; Gjedde, A.; Samson, F.E.: Neuroanatomical functional mapping by the radioactive 2-deoxy-*D*-glucose method. Neurosci. Res. Program Bull. *14:* 457–518 (1976).

9 Poggio, T.; Reichardt, W.: Visual control of orientation behaviour in the fly. II. Toward the underlying neural interactions. Q. Rev. Biophys. *9:* 377–438 (1976).

10 Reichardt, W.; Poggio, T.: Visual control of orientation behaviour in the fly. I. A quantitative analysis. Q. Rev. Biophys. *9:* 311–375 (1976).

11 Sokoloff, L.; Reivich, M; Kennedy, C.; Des Rosiers, M.H.; Patlak, C.S.; Pettigrew, K.D.; Sakurada, O.; Shinohara, M.: The ^{14}C-deoxyglucose method for the measurement of local cerebral glucose utilization: theory, procedure, and normal values in the conscious and anesthetized albino rat. J. Neurochem. *28:* 897–916 (1977).

12 Strausfeld, N.J.: Atlas of an insect brain (Springer, Berlin 1976).

13 Wenzl, H.: Die Verwertung von Glukose und Fruktose im Ruhestoffwechsel von *Calliphora erythrocephala.* Z. vergl. Physiol. *65:* 340–350 (1969).

Dr. E. Buchner, Max-Planck-Institut für biologische Kybernetik, Spemannstrasse 38, D-7400 Tübingen (FRG)

Eur. Neurol. *20:* 157–161 (1981)

High Resolution Radioautographic Study of the Inner Ear following in vivo Tritiated Deoxyglucose Administration[1]

R. Pujol, A. Sans, A. Calas[2]

Université de Provence et CNRS, Marseille, et Université des Sciences et Techniques du Languedoc, Montpellier, France

Key Words. ^{3}H-DG in vivo administration · Light and EM radioautography · Vestibular and cochlear metabolism

Abstract. Light and high resolution radioautography were performed on cat and guinea pig inner ear after an in vivo administration of tritiated deoxyglucose and conventional histological treatments. In the guinea pig cochlea a diffuse radioautographic reaction product appeared on all the neurosensory and surrounding structures, with a more intense labelling of stria vascularis and Reissner's membrane. In the cat vestibular organ a diffuse reaction was also noted, with an intense clear-cut labelling of some dark cells at the base of the lateral crista and on some cells limiting the endolymphatic space, opposite the utricular macula. At the EM level, the silver grain distribution preferentially appeared to be localized on the cytoplasmic glycogen granules. In addition, some sensory cells were densely marked, the silver grains neither occurring on the nucleus nor on the surrounding nerve calyx, and rarely upon the mitochondria. These data indicate that using classical histological treatments, it is possible to retain a part of the radioactive molecules around the injection site. The possible physiological meaning of the selective labelling of some cellular and subcellular compartments is discussed.

Introduction

The ^{14}C-deoxyglucose (DG) method has been used as a biochemical [14] or as a morpho-functional [10] qualitative tool in studies of various sensory systems [7, 13, 16]. The corresponding sensory organs have been studied less owing mainly to the low resolution of that method. Lower energy isotopes, like ^{3}H might improve this shortcoming. But using the cryostat-stripping film technique, to retain in situ labelled molecules like ^{3}H-DG, the tissue preservation is poor and the observation limited at the histological level [9]. A complex histological processing by perfusion of all fixation, dehydration and embedding

1 Supported by grants from CNRS (ERA 537, ATP 79), Inserm (ATP 81–79–113) and DGRST (Dyn. neur.-BRD).

2 We thank *E. Carlier, M. Chat* and *C. Devigne* for technical assistance, and *A. Shnerson* for correcting the manuscript.

products has been recently proposed by *Des Rosiers and Descarries* [4] in order to allow a radioautographic study with the dipping technique. In this case, the labelling is qualitatively comparable to that with ^{14}C-DG cryostat technique. We used this method in the cochlea and on semi-thin plastic embedded sections, a diffuse distribution of silver grains occurred on all the structures, but with a more intense labelling of the stria vascularis and Reissner's membrane [2].

In another sensory organ, the fish retina, it has been more recently shown that in vitro incubation in ^{3}H-DG followed by conventional fixation and embedding procedures leads to a differential radioautographic labelling of the retinal structures which depend on dark or light experimental conditions [1]. The present work aimed to investigate, by light [12] and high-resolution radioautography, the labelling of the two sensory organs of the inner ear – cochlea and vestibule – after an in vivo administration of ^{3}H-DG and conventional histological treatments.

Material and Methods

In 2 adult Nembutal-anesthetized cats, 0.4 μl of artificial endolymph containing 10 μCi/μl of ^{3}H-DG (Amersham, 19 Ci/mmol) was directly injected into the lateral canal and 4 μl was pipetted into the vestibule through the oval window. Brief ampulopetal stimulations [3] of the left crista ampullaris were performed during 20 min at a rate of 4/min.

In 2 adult Pentothal-anesthetized guinea pigs, 10 μl of artificial perilymph containing 10 μCi/μl of ^{3}H-DG was injected into the first coil of the tympanic scala. During the 10-min injection period and for the next 20 min, the subjects were exposed in free-field to a tone (6–12 kHz, 100 dB SPL). In both types of experiments, sensory organs were fixed in situ by a small volume of 2.5% glutaraldehyde in 0.15 *M* phosphate buffer. Vestibular and cochlear tissues were immersed for 30 min in the same fixative, postfixed with osmium tetroxide, dehydrated in ethanol and embedded in Epon. Semi-thin sections were radioautographed by dipping into K5 Ilford nuclear emulsion exposed for 15–40 days, before being developed in D19B Kodak. Thin sections were radioautographed with L4 Ilford nuclear emulsion and exposed for 40–60 days before developing with Microdol × Kodak [8].

Results

Cochlea

A diffuse radioautographic reaction consisting in a profuse nonselective distribution of silver grains occurred in all the cochlear structures. However, a clear-cut more intense labelling was seen especially on the stria vascularis (fig. 1), and on Reissner's membrane.

Vestibule

A diffuse radioautographic reaction occurred upon all the vestibular structures surrounding the injection sites. Several types of structures were more intensely labelled. Distinct accumulations of silver grains occurred on the base of the ampular crista and on some

Fig. 1. Radioautograph of semi-thin section of the cochlea. An intense labelling is seen on the whole stria vascularis (limited by the two arrows). Note the contrast with the diffuse labelling on surrounding structures. × 650.

Fig. 2, 4. Radioautographs of semi-thin **(2)** or thin **(4)** sections of the utricular macula. The perikaryon of some type-I sensory cells is densely labelled. The silver grains spare the nucleus and the surrounding nerve calyx; they are scarce upon mitchondria. **2** × 1,800. **4** × 12,000.

Fig. 3. Radioautograph of thin section of the epithelium limiting the endolymphatic space, opposite the macula. In the intensely labelled cell (arrows), as well as in the neighbouring ones, silver grains preferentially overlaid glycogen. × 8,000.

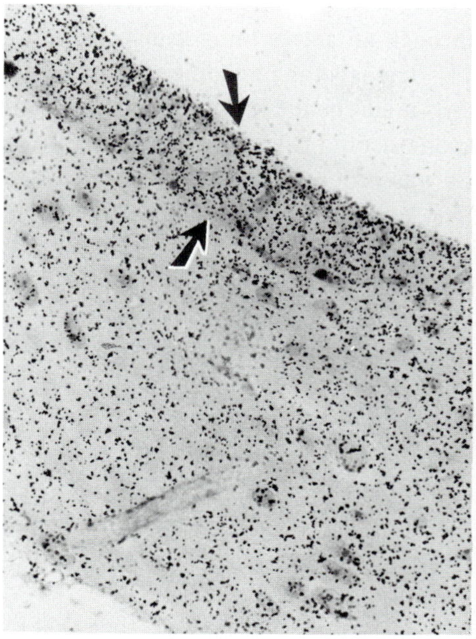
1

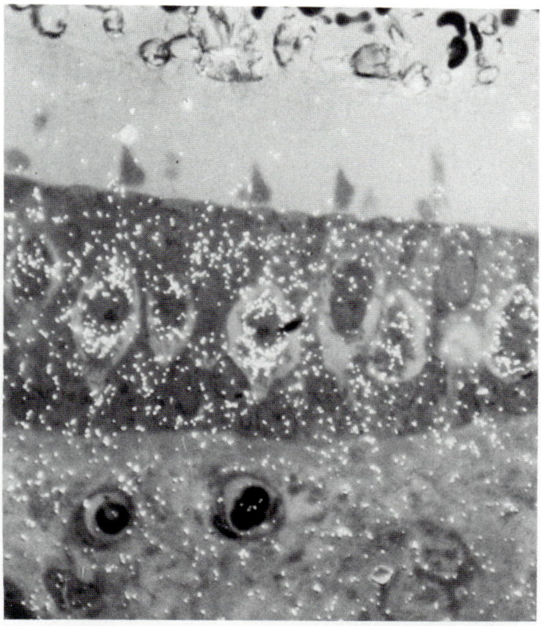
2

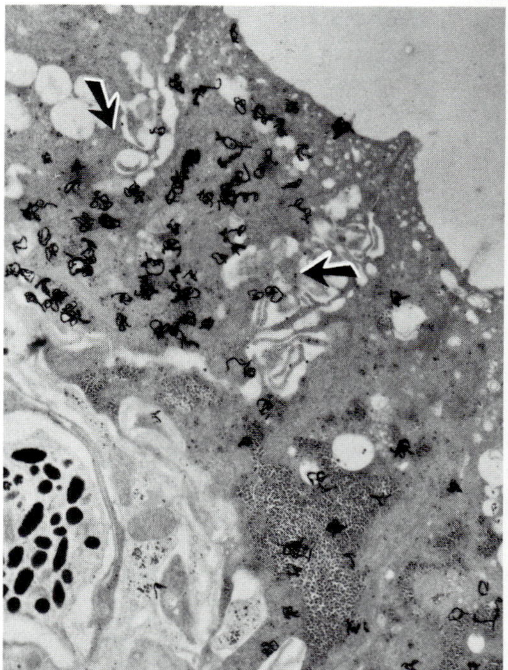
3

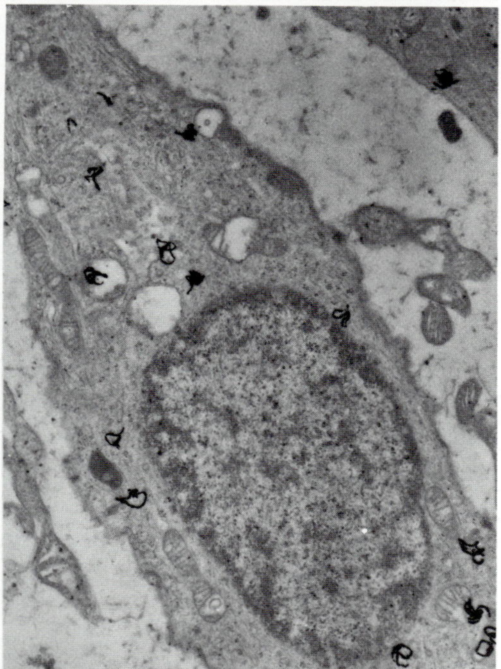
4

epithelial cells limiting the endolymphatic space opposite the macula. Moreover, clusters of silver grains overlaid the perikaryon of some of the type I sensory cells in the utricular macula (fig. 2) and lateral ampulla. At the electron microscopic level some epithelial dark cells were conspicuously labelled; silver grains being preferentially located on the glycogen (fig. 3). In the labelled sensory cells silver grains never occurred on the nucleus or on the surrounding nerve calyx; they were scarce upon mitochondria (fig. 4).

Discussion

It is known that within short survival times, the metabolism of 2-DG in brain cells is restricted to its phosphorylation into 2-DG-6-phosphate [14]. Our results show that a portion of these molecules can be retained near the injection site after conventional fixation, dehydration and embedding procedures. The stria vascularis labelling is similar after the present treatment and earlier described one [2] using the perfusion processing where good tracer retention was demonstrated [4]. This suggests that the radioactive patterns correspond to a low displacement of the labelled molecules. Trapped molecules might correspond to protein or glycogen-bound ^{3}H-DG – ^{3}H-DGP. The present method is simpler and easier than the perfusion processing, it allows similar good tissue preservation and it permits high resolution radioautographic study.

In both inner ear sensory organs, the prominent labelling of Reissner's membrane, stria vascularis and vestibular dark cells seems to correspond to a high glucidic metabolism. Actually, such structures are implied in producing and maintaining endolymph through an active ionic transportation [5, 6, 11]. The labelling of some sensory vestibular cells might be the result of their stimulated or spontaneous [15] activity. A similar hypothesis was proposed to explain the in vitro ^{3}H-DG labelling of some retinal receptors [1]. Our ultrastructural data regarding the lack of nuclear labelling confirms the low displacement of the tracer. Moreover, they suggest that this in vivo method can be used in some models to study the metabolic activity at cellular and even subcellular levels.

References

1 Basinger, S.F.; Gordon, W.C.; Lam, D.M.K.: Differential labelling of retinal neurons by ^{3}H-2-deoxyglucose. Nature, Lond. *280:* 682–683 (1979).

2 Calas, A.; Orsini, J.C.; Dusticier, G.; Cooper, H.; Carlier, E.; Pujol, R.: Distribution de la radioactivité dans le tissu nerveux après administration de désoxyglucose tritié. Etude radioautographique chez le rat. J. Physiol., Paris *75:* 47A (1979).

3 Dechesne, C.; Sans, A.: A new stimulation technique of the crista ampullaris of the lateral canal in the adult cat; study of the action potential of the vestibular nerve. Experientia *35:* 846–847 (1979).

4 Des Rosiers, M.H.; Descarries, L.: Adaptation de la méthode au désoxyglucose à l'échelle cellulaire: préparation histologique du système nerveux central en vue de la radioautographie à haute résolution. C.r. hebd. Séanc. Acad. Sci., Paris, sér. D *287:* 153–154 (1978).

5 Dohlman, G.F.: Histochemistry and metabolism of the inner ear; in Kornhuber, Handbook of sensory physiology. Part I. Vestibular system, vol. 6, pp. 185–212 (Springer, Berlin 1974).

6 Hinojosa, R.; Rodriguez-Echandia, E.L.: The fine structure of the stria vascularis of the cat inner ear. Am. J. Anat. *118:* 631–664 (1966).

7 Hubel, D.H.; Wiesel, T.N.; Stryker, M.P.: Orientation columns in macaque monkey visual cortex demonstrated by the 2-deoxyglucose autoradiographic technique. Nature, Lond. *269:* 328–330 (1977).

8 Larra, F.; Droz, B.: Techniques radioautographiques et leur application à l'étude du renouvellement des constituants cellulaires. J. Microscopie *9:* 845–880 (1970).

9 Lippe, W.R.; Steward, O.; Rubel, E.: The effect of unilateral basilar papilla removal upon nuclei laminaris and magnocellularis of the chick examined with ^{3}H-2-deoxy-*D*-glucose autoradiography. Brain Res. *196:* 43–58 (1980).

10 Plum, F.; Djedde, A.; Samson, F.E.: Neuroanatomical functional mapping by the radioactive 2-deoxy-*D*-glucose method. Neurosci. Res. Prog. Bull. *14:* 457–518 (1976).

11 Ross, M.D.: Glycogen accumulation in Reissner's membrane following chemical sympathectomy with 6-hydroxydopamine. Acta otolar. *86:* 314–330 (1978).

12 Sans, A.; Pujol, R.; Carlier, E.; Calas, A.: Détection cellulaire de l'incorporation in vivo de 2-désoxyglucose tritié. Etude radioautographique dans l'oreille interne. C.r. hebd. Séanc. Acad. Sci., Paris, sér. D *290:* 1225–1227 (1980).

13 Skeen, L.C.: Odor-induced patterns of deoxyglucose consumption in the olfactory bulb of the tree shrew, *Tupaia glis.* Brain Res. *124:* 147–153 (1977).

14 Sokoloff, L.; Reivich, M.; Kennedy, C.; Des Rosiers, M.H.; Patlak, C.S.; Pettigrew, K.D.; Sakurada, O.; Shinohara, M.: The ^{14}C-deoxyglucose method for the measurement of local cerebral glucose utilisation: theory, procedure, and normal values in the conscious and anesthetized albino rat. J. Neurochem. *28:* 891–916 (1977).

15 Walsh, B.T.; Miller, J.B.; Gacek, P.R.; Kiang, N.Y.S.: Spontaneous activity in the eighth cranial nerve of the cat. Int. J. Neurosci. *3:* 221–236 (1972).

16 Webster, W.R.; Serviere, J.; Batini, C.; Laplante, S.: Autoradiographic demonstration with 2-^{14}C-deoxyglucose of frequency selectivity in the auditory system of the cat under conditions of functional activity. Neurosci. Lett. *10:* 43–48 (1978).

Prof. R. Pujol, Laboratoire de Neurophysiologie sensorielle, Université de Provence, Centre de St-Jérôme, F-13397 Marseille, Cédex 4 (France)

Eur. Neurol. *20:* 162–168 (1981)

Local Cerebral Glucose Utilization in the Newborn Brain

N. Grégoire, R. Pontier, G. Salamon

Laboratoire de Biochimie et Circulation Cérébrale, Service du Professeur G. Salamon, CHU La Timone, Marseille, France

Key Words. ^{14}C-2-DG · Regional cerebral energy metabolism · Newborn brain · Pattern of metabolic needs · Transient asphyxia

Abstract. Local cerebral glucose utilization (LCGU) was determined in 2- to 8-day-old beagle dogs by the quantitative ^{14}C-deoxyglucose autoradiographic method. In physiologically controlled puppies (BP 66 ± 3 mm Hg; paO_2 71 ± 2 mm Hg; $paCO_2$ 35 mm Hg, pH 7.39 ± 0.04; hematocrit 39 ± 2%), the 2-deoxyglucose (2-DG) autoradiographs and quantitative data reveal a characteristic pattern of regional energy metabolic needs in the normal newborn brain: highest glucose consumption values are found in brain stem nuclei (inferior olivary nucleus 19 ± 4 μmol/100 g/min; vestibular nucleus 26 ± 5; red nucleus 15 ± 2) and in selected deep cerebral structures (subthalamic nucleus 18 ± 4; ventrolateral thalamic nucleus 12 ± 2, ...) whereas consistently relative lower glucose consumption is found in the cerebral cortex (mean 7 ± 1). This data is in agreement with local cerebral blood flow studies in the newborn puppy. A characteristic functional anatomy of the newborn dog brain is demonstrated. The value of 0.558 ± 0.031 for the lumped constant was used in the calculation of LCGU. In puppies previously asphyxiated for 2.5–3.5 min 1–2 days prior to the 2-DG procedure, no significant effect upon regional metabolism was demonstrated.

Whole brain energy metabolism studies have pointed out the low metabolic demands of the newborn brain, compared to the adult [*Himwich and Fazekas,* 1941; *Thurston and McDougal,* 1969; *Duffy* et al., 1975; *Purves and James,* 1969; *Grégoire* et al., 1978].

Recent studies of local cerebral blood flow by *Kennedy* et al. [1971, 1972] have shown higher rates of perfusion in selected deep cerebral structures and brain stem nuclei than in the cerebral cortex; this suggested a more active local tissue energy metabolism in these areas.

The ^{14}C-2-deoxyglucose (^{14}C-2-DG) autoradiographic method for determining local cerebral glucose utilization (LCGU) of *Soko-*

loff et al. [1977] gave us the opportunity to characterize the regional aspects of neonatal energy metabolism and to quantitate glucose consumption of various structures of the newborn brain. We measured local cerebral glucose consumption by the ^{14}C-2-DG autoradiographic technique, on the same experimental model as in a previous study of newborn whole brain metabolism in the beagle dog [*Grégoire* et al., 1978].

The normal pattern of regional glucose consumption in the newborn dog brain is determined. This confirms a striking heterogeneity of cerebral metabolic needs in gray matter structures at this age.

Material and Methods

Studies were performed on newborn, pure-bred beagle dogs, 2–8 days old. The dogs were nourished by the mother up to the time of experimentation. The animals were obtained with the pregnant mothers, 2 weeks prior to the time of birth, from EVIC-CEBA farms.

Local cerebral glucose utilization was determined by the quantitative ^{14}C-2-DG method [*Sokoloff* et al., 1977] based on the injection of a radioactive tracer for glucose metabolism: 1-^{14}C-2-DG and a quantitative autoradiographic procedure to measure ^{14}C local concentration in various structures of the brain.

Experimental Procedure

The experimental procedure is outlined in table I.

Prior to the acute ^{14}C-2-DG experiment all animals were intubated with a 'VYGON' endotracheal tube (25–30 mm OD) for the anesthesia and catheterization procedures. Heart rate and blood pressure were continuously monitored by a non-invasive oscillometric method (DINAMAP) during anesthesia.

Conditions

The experimental procedure to measure local cerebral glucose utilization was performed on two groups of newborn dogs: (1) control group, 4 normal newborn dogs, without any previous treatment; (2) post-asphyxia group: 2 newborn dogs treated as follows: 24 or 48 h prior to the 2-DG experiment asphyxia was induced by clamping of the endotracheal tube for 2.5 min (animal No. 1) and 3.5 min (animal No. 2) until gasping and cardiovascular insufficiency were observed, at this time the animals were ressuscitated with a return of normal blood pressure and heart rate; dogs given back to the mother to be nourished normally; 2-DG procedure performed 1 or 2 days later, exactly as in the control group.

Calculations

Rates of local cerebral glucose utilization were calculated from the brain concentration of ^{14}C (derived from its optical density and calibration curve of ^{14}C standards) and from the plasma concentrations of ^{14}C-2-DG and glucose according to the equation developed by *Sokoloff* et al. [1977]. This defines LCGU in terms of measurable variables and definable constants. Of these constants, the 'lumped constant' is the most important and has been shown to vary with the species. The lumped constant in the puppy has been previously assessed by us and *Duffy* et al. [1979] and was found to be equal to 0.558 ± 0.031.

Table I. Experimental procedure for local cerebral glucose utilization measurement

1 Physiological study
2 Anesthesia and surgical procedures
3 ^{14}C-2-deoxyglucose acute experiment
4 Sectioning of frozen brain
5 Quantitative autoradiography
6 Computerized calculation of glucose consumption
7 Pathology

Table II. Physiological conditions of the animals (means ± SEM)

Arterial mean blood pressure	66 ± 3 mm Hg
Arterial blood gases	
paO_2	71 ± 2 mm Hg
$paCO_2$	35 ± 1 mm Hg
pH	7.39 ± 0.035
Hematocrit	39 ± 2%

1

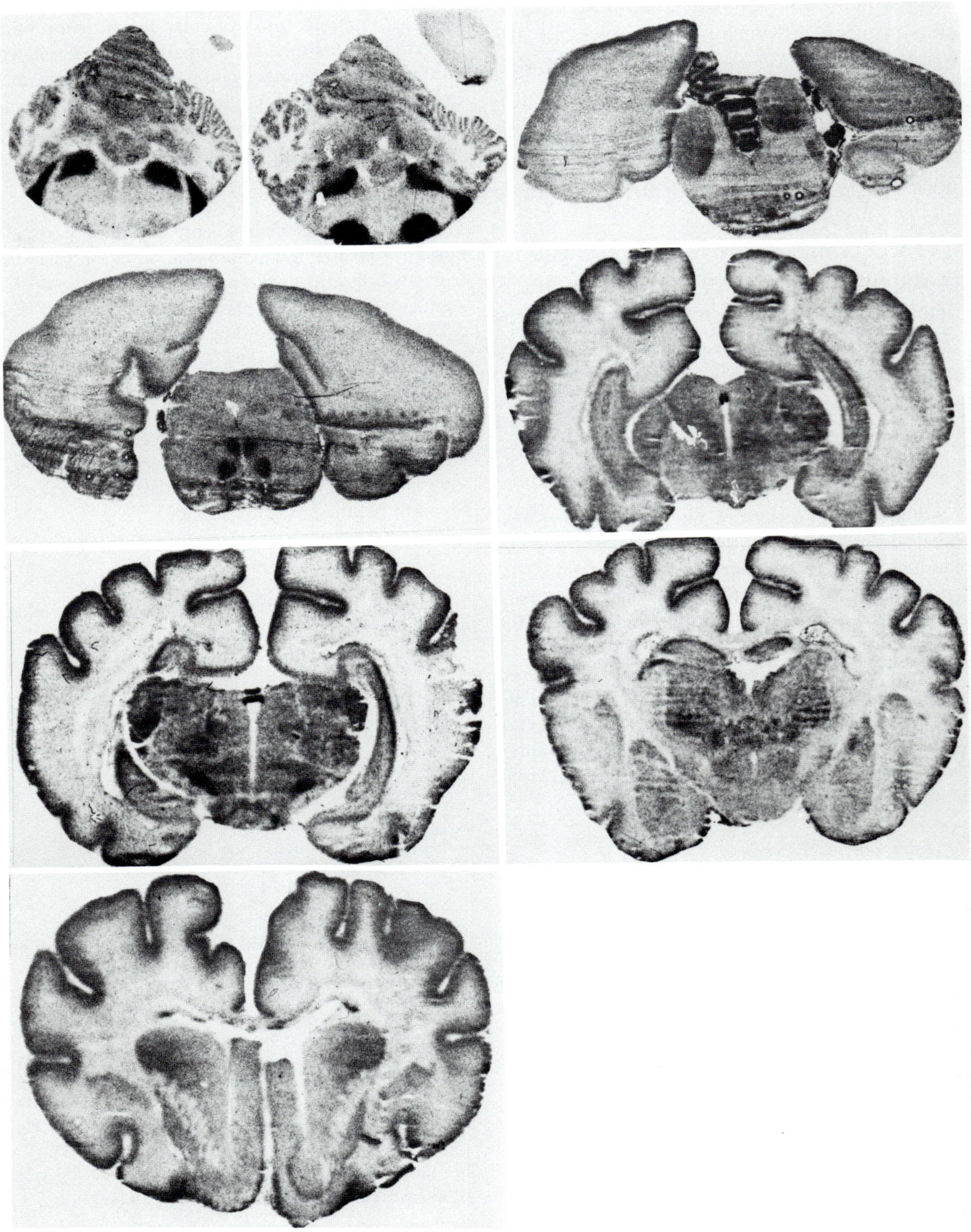

2

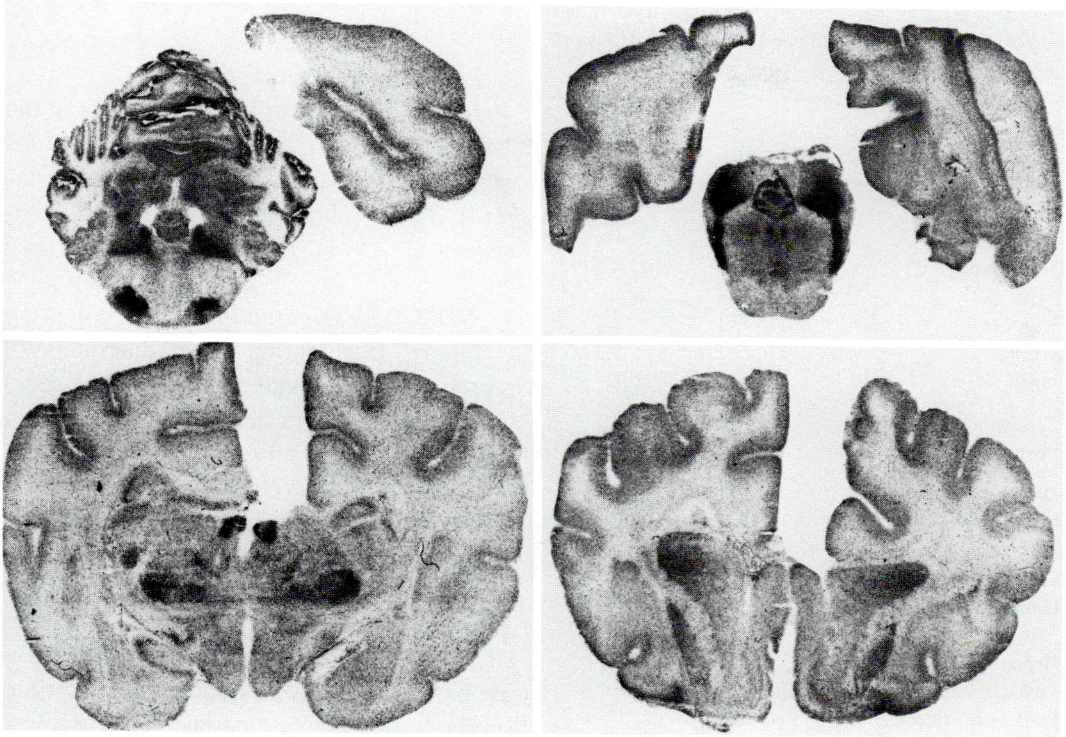

a b c d

Fig. 1. Representative autoradiographs of various coronal sections of newborn dog brain from the control group. Relatively high metabolic rates shown by dark regions. **a** Medulla (upper part): high activity dorsally in vestibular nuclei and laterally in cochlear nuclei. Cerebellum cortex, white matter, dentate nuclei laterally and vermian nuclei on the midline. **b** Pontine section: ventrally the superior olivar nucleus and dorsally the vestibular nucleus are very dark. **c** Lower midbrain: inferior colliculi very marked compared to the occipital cortex. **d** Upper midbrain: oculomotor nuclei medially and red nuclei are laterally easily distinguishable. **e** Diencephalon (caudal aspect): medial geniculate bodies laterally; pulvinar and habenular nuclei medially. Temporal lobe: hippocampus medially and piriform and auditive cortex laterally. Parietal cortex in the upper part of the section. **f** Diencephalon (central aspect): ventrally subthalamic nuclei, dorsally, lateral geniculate bodies very dense compared to the cerebral cortex. **g** Diencephalon (rostral aspect): the ventrolateral thalamic nucleus is very dense compared to the hypothalamic region. Laterally, amygdala in the temporal lobe. **h** Frontal section through the basal ganglia: caudate nucleus medially, lenticular nucleus laterally both are dense compared to the anterior limb of the internal capsule.

Fig. 2. Representative 2-DG autoradiographs of coronal sections of newborn dog brain from the post transient asphyxia group. **a** Pontine section: superior olivary nucleus and vestibular nucleus. **b** Lower midbrain: inferior colliculi contrasting with the occipital cortex. **c** Diencephalon: habenular nuclei ventro-postero-lateral thalamic nuclei: very high metabolic activity compared to the cerebral cortex. **d** Frontal section through the basal ganglia: caudate and lenticular nuclei.

Table III. Local cerebral glucose utilization: values in the normal newborn dog and 48 h after a transient asphyxia (µmol/100 g/min; mean ± SEM)

Structure	Normal group	Post-asphyxia group
Cerebral cortex		
Occipital	6 ± 1	8 ± 1
Temporal	6 ± 1	6 ± 1
Parietal	7 ± 1	6 ± 1
Sensorimotor	8 ± 1	9 ± 2
Frontal	6 ± 1	5 ± 1
Mean	7 ± 1	7 ± 1
Cerebellum		
Cortex	13 ± 2	12 ± 3
Deep cerebral		
Medial geniculate	8 ± 1	12 ± 2
Lateral geniculate	13 ± 2	14 ± 2
Subthalamic nucleus	18 ± 4	17 ± 4
Habenular nucleus	15 ± 3	17 ± 4
Amygdala	6 ± 1	5 ± 1
Hippocampus	7 ± 1	
Caudate nucleus	8 ± 1	14 ± 3
Lentiform nucleus	8 ± 1	
Thalamus, ventrolateral	12 ± 2	
Hypothalamus	4 ± 0	
Brain stem		
Inferior olivary nucleus	19 ± 4	17 ± 2
Vestibular nucleus	26 ± 5	44 ± 6
Cochlear nucleus	30 ± 6	32 ± 7
Superior colliculus	8 ± 1	9 ± 1
Inferior colliculus	31 ± 6	42 ± 8
Red nucleus	15 ± 2	
Oculomotor nuclei	15 ± 1	
White matter		
Mean	3 ± 0	

Results

Physiological Parameters

Just prior to and at the termination of the 2-DG experiment, physiological conditions were assessed. Mean values are listed in table II. These values agree with those of *Kennedy* et al. [1971].

2-DG Autoradiographs

Figure 1a–h shows autoradiographs of representative coronal sections of the newborn dog brain from the control group. They provide a pictorial representation of the relative rates of glucose consumption in the various cerebral structures of the newborn dog brain: white matter (fig. 1a, h) being characterized by a low optical density and, conversely, gray matter by a relatively high density. This mapping technique reveals a striking pattern of regional glucose consumption: cerebral cortical areas demonstrate a very low metabolic activity compared to central gray matter (fig. 1e–h) and brain stem nuclei (fig. 1a–d). This pattern is not found in adult brains of the rat or monkey, in which the cerebral cortex appears to have a much higher density.

In the animals previously asphyxiated, 2-DG autoradiographs (fig. 2a–d) show the same mapping of regional cerebral glucose metabolism as in the control group.

Quantitative Data

Values of local cerebral glucose consumption measured in 27 various structures are listed in table III. The quantitative data seem to show low metabolic rates of glucose consumption similar to results obtained in whole brain studies [*Grégoire* et al., 1978].

A lower metabolic rate of glucose consumption is found in white matter compared to gray matter. In addition, the LCGU values within the gray matter are heterogenous: higher rates of glucose consumption in brain stem nuclei and various central gray structures compared to consistently lower values in cortical gray areas.

LCGU values in the post-transient asphyxia are not significantly different from those of the control group.

Discussion

Our data on local energy metabolism of the newborn dog brain are in agreement with local cerebral blood flow studies in puppies of similar age by *Kennedy* et al. [1971, 1972]. They are also consistent with studies of in vitro oxygen consumption by *Himwich and Fazekas* [1941].

A variety of applications of the ^{14}C-2-DG method have extensively shown a clear relationship between local cerebral functional activity and glucose consumption [*Sokoloff,* 1977]. Therefore the present study provides a functional anatomy of the newborn dog brain. This functional anatomy differs from that of the adult: the neocortex being less active than phylogenetically older parts of the brain in the neonate. This probably reflects differences of maturation in the nervous system of the dog at this age.

The present findings of a particular high metabolic activity in brain stem nuclei and some diencephalic structures, may also explain the anatomico-pathological damages secondary to experimental asphyxia [*Jilek* et al., 1964; *Myers,* 1972].

This study failed to detect any regional energy metabolic effect in the post-transient asphyxia group. This is in keeping with data of *Siesjo and Plum* [1972] on cerebral energy balance after short-term asphyxia. Nevertheless, it is possible that, with longer periods of asphyxia, the results will be different.

Conclusions

The present study provides a functional anatomy of the newborn brain of the dog, with a characteristic pattern of regional energy metabolism: higher glucose consumption rates in brain stem nuclei and various deep cerebral structures, and consistently lower metabolic rates in the cerebral cortex. This differs from results found in adult brains of the rat or monkey.

Quantitative data of LCGU confirm these differences and the low metabolic rates of glucose consumption, compared to the adult whole-brain glucose consumption.

Quantification is required to affirm regional metabolic effects of pathological conditions. We plan to continue the post-asphyxia LCGU studies after longer periods of asphyxia.

Acknowledgement

The authors gratefully acknowledge the technical assistance of Mrs. *M. Morel* and Mr. *J.M. Corbaz* (Inserm U-S Marseille).

This work was supported by a grant of Inserm (CRL).

References

Duffy, T.E.; Cavazzuti, M.; Grégoire, N.M.; Cruz, N.F.; Kennedy, C.; Sokoloff, L.: Regional cerebral glucose metabolism in newborn beagle dogs. Trans. Am. Soc. Neurochem. *10:* 171 (1979).

Duffy, T.E.; Kohle, S.J.; Vannucci, R.C.: Carbohydrate and energy metabolism in perinatal rat brain: relation to survival in anoxia. J. Neurochem. (1975).

Grégoire, N.M.; Gjedde, A.; Plum, F.; Duffy, T.E.: Cerebral blood flow and cerebral metabolic rates for oxygen, glucose and ketone bodies in newborn dog. J. Neurochem. *30:* 63–69 (1978).

Himwich, H.E.; Fazekas, J.F.: Comparative studies of the metabolism of the brain of infant and adult dogs. Am. J. Physiol. *132:* 454–458 (1941).

Jilek, L.; Fischer, J.; Krulich, L.; Trojan, S.: The reaction of the brain to stagnant hypoxia and anoxia during ontogeny. Prog. Brain Res. *9:* 113–131 (1964).

Kennedy, C.; Grave, G.D.; Jehle, J.W.: Effect of hyperoxia on the cerebral circulation of the newborn puppy. Pediat. Res. *5:* 659–667 (1971).

Kennedy, C.; Grave, G.D.; Jehle, J.W.; Sokoloff, L.: Changes in blood flow in the component structures of the dog brain during postnatal maturation. J. Neurochem. *19:* 2423–2433 (1972).

Myers, R.E.: Two patterns of perinatal brain damage and their conditions of occurrence. Am. J. Obstet. Gynec. *112:* 246–276 (1972).

Purves, M.J.; James, I.M.: Observations on the control of cerebral blood flow in the sheep fetus and newborn lamb. Circulation Res. *25:* 651–667 (1969).

Siesjo, B.K.; Plum, F.: Pathophysiology of anoxia brain damage; in Gaull, Biology of brain dysfunction, vol. 1, pp. 319–372 (Plenum Press, New York 1972).

Sokoloff, L.: Relation between physiological function and energy metabolism in the central nervous system. J. Neurochem. *29:* 13–26 (1977).

Sokoloff, L.; Reivich, M.; Kennedy, C.; Des Rosiers, M.M.; Patlak, C.S.; Pettigrew, K.D.; Sakurada, O.; Shinohara, M.: The ^{14}C deoxyglucose method for the measurement of local cerebral glucose utilization. Theory, procedure and normal values in the conscious and anesthetized albino rat. J. Neurochem. *28:* 897–916 (1977).

Thurston, J.H.; McDougal, D.B., Jr.: Effect of ischemia on metabolism of the brain of the newborn mouse. Am. J. Physiol. *216:* 348–352 (1969).

Tyler, D.B.; Harreveld, A. van: The respiration of the developing brain. Am. J. Physiol. *136:* 600–603 (1942).

Vannucci, R.C.; Duffy, T.E.: Cerebral metabolism in newborn dogs during reversible asphyxia. Ann. Neurol. *1:* 528–534 (1977).

Dr. Nicole Grégoire, Laboratoire de Biochimie et Circulation Cérébrale, Service du Professeur G. Salamon, CHU La Timone, F-13385 Marseille (France)

Eur. Neurol. *20:* 169–172 (1981)

Application of the 2-Deoxy-*D*-[^{14}C]-Glucose Method to the Mouse for Measuring Local Cerebral Glucose Utilization[1]

T. Nowaczyk[a], *M.H. Des Rosiers*[b]

[a] Inserm U-52, Université Claude-Bernard, Lyon, France; [b] Université de Montréal, Départment de Physiologie, Montréal, Québec, Canada

Key Words. [^{14}C]-Deoxyglucose · Cerebral · Glucose · Utilization · Mouse

Abstract. The 2-deoxy-*D*-[^{14}C]-glucose method for the quantitative determination of local cerebral glucose utilization has been applied to the mouse. The experiments were conducted in awake freely moving animals. Local cerebral glucose utilization was found to vary widely throughout the brain with the lowest values in white matter and the highest in gray matter. The most metabolically active structures were those involved in auditory function or in general motor activity. All the values were lower than those observed previously in the conscious rat. The use of free-moving animals may be of importance since it allows the study of physiological or pathological behavioral states.

Introduction

The 2-deoxy-*D*-[^{14}C]-glucose ([^{14}C]-DG) method initially described by *Sokoloff* et al. [8] represents one of the best available tools for measuring local cerebral glucose utilization (LCGU) and it has been used for such determinations in some mammalian species [4, 8]. Our choice of the mouse, for which no LCGU data are available, is essentially justified by the existence in this species of a number of inbred strains of neurological mutants [7] and by the possibility that metabolic studies could give new insights on some of the central phenomena linked to or involved in their abnormalities. In this paper we shall report on preliminary experiments realized in mice, with special emphasis on the methodological problems encountered in adapting the classical procedure of *Sokoloff* et al. [8].

[1] This work was supported by Inserm (U-52), CNRS (LA 162) and DRET (78–82) and realized within France-Quebec cooperation.

Material and Methods

Inbred female mice from the C57BL6 strain, (20 g each) were submitted to one of the following two surgical procedures.

Under light halothane anesthesia, catheterization of the femoral vein and artery was performed in 4 mice which were lightly restrained for a further 24-hour period (plaster cast).

4 other mice were cannulated in the common carotid artery on one side and the jugular vein on the opposite side. The catheters were threaded subcutaneously onto the skull where they were fixed in order to allow free activity. After recovery from anesthesia, the mice were replaced in their usual environment (food and water ad libitum; light/dark: 12 h/12 h with light on at 7 a.m.; temperature 24 ± 2 °C) during a 24-hour period.

In both groups the classical procedure described by *Sokoloff* et al. [8] was applied. At 1 p.m., a pulse of 3 μCi of [14C]-DG (specific activity 53 mCi/mmol: New England Nuclear Corp., Boston, Mass.) in 15 μl of saline was injected through the venous catheter. Timed arterial blood samples of 30 μl each were collected during the ensuing 45-min period, and used for the determinations of [14C]-DG (4 μl; liquid scintillation counter) and plasma glucose concentrations (5 μl; glucose oxidase method) (fig. 1). The animals were sacrificed 45 min after the [14C]-DG administration and their brains rapidly removed and frozen in liquid nitrogen. The autoradiographs were obtained from serial brain sections (20 μm) exposed during a 7-day period [6].

The LCGU was calculated in various structures using a Leitz MPV microscope photometer (compact model) and the operational equation [8]. The constants for transport and phosphorylation and the lumped constant were those measured in the rat.

Arterial blood pressure, hematocrit, arterial blood pH, PCO_2, PO_2 were also measured during the experiment and, in 1 mouse, the bilateral cortical activity was recorded through electrodes chronically implanted before catheterization.

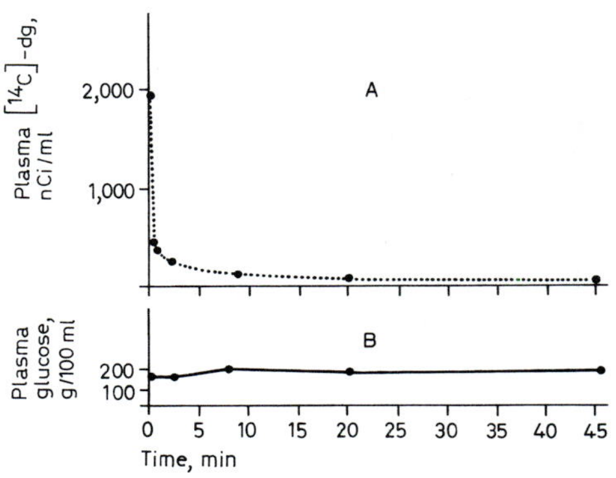

Fig. 1. Arterial plasma [14C]-deoxyglucose **(A)** and glucose **(B)** concentrations from the administration of a tracer pulse to sacrifice.

Results

All the mice with femoral cannulation and relative restraint were hyperglycemic at the time of the [14C]-DG experiment (more than 2 g/l). Due to the influence of this parameter on [14C]-DG uptake, these animals were not used for LCGU determinations.

In the free-moving mice with carotid and jugular cannulations, glycemia was within the normal range, as were the other measured physiological variables (arterial PO_2, PCO_2 and pH, hematocrit and mean arterial blood pressure), allowing the utilization of the [14C]-DG method (fig. 1).

A typical autoradiographic pattern of glucose utilization is shown in figure 2 where, at the level of the pons and cerebellum, a high rate of metabolic activity is obvious in the cochlear, vestibular and cerebellar nuclei.

Some of the quantitative data from those obtained from 50 different brain structures are expressed in table I. The LCGU is low and homogeneous in white matter (average value: 24 $\mu mol \cdot 100\, g^{-1} \cdot min^{-1}$). In gray matter, the values vary from 30 $\mu mol \cdot 100\, g^{-1} \cdot min^{-1}$ in the hypothalamic area to 122 $\mu mol \cdot 100\, g^{-1} \cdot min^{-1}$ in the inferior colliculus. The ratio of LCGU in gray matter to that in white matter was 2.33.

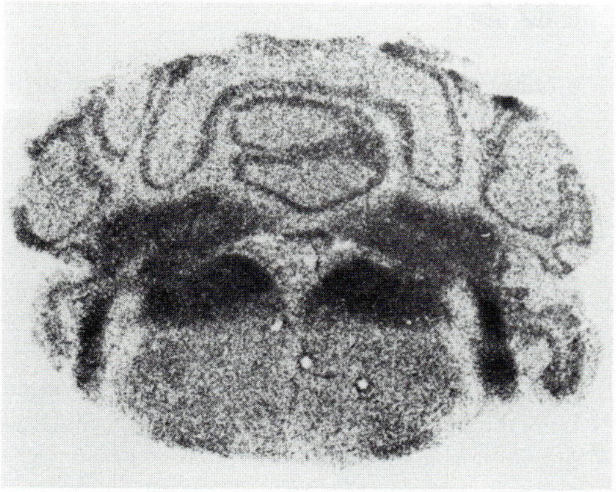

Fig. 2. [^{14}C]-deoxyglucose autoradiograph of a coronal brain section from a C57BL6 mouse at the level of the pons and cerebellum. Note the high metabolic rate, marked by dark regions, in vestibular, cochlear and cerebellar nuclei. The dark band in the cerebellum corresponds to the granular layer.

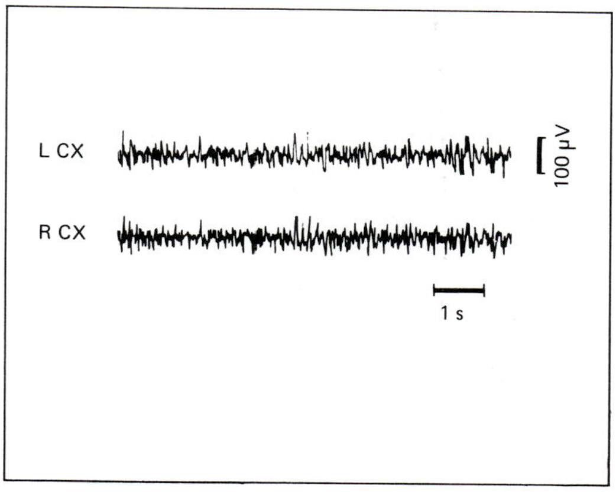

Fig. 3. Right (R CX) and left (L CX) fronto-parietal electrocorticograms recorded 24 h after recovery from carotid artery and jugular vein catheterization.

Table I. Local cerebral glucose utilization in the free-moving C57BL6 mouse

Structure	Value µmol/100 g/min
Gray matter	
Visual cortex	53 ± 5
Auditory cortex	73 ± 6
Mammillary body	81 ± 5
Interpeduncular nucleus	81 ± 3
Inferior colliculus	122 ± 12
Superior olive	68 ± 8
Cerebellar nuclei	64 ± 2
Vestibular nuclei	86 ± 2
Cochlear	
ventral nucleus	50 ± 2
dorsal nucleus	72 ± 5
Inferior olive	
dorsal nucleus	49 ± 3
median nucleus	53 ± 4
White matter	
Anterior commissure	24 ± 3
Corpus callosum	25 ± 4
Internal capsule	19 ± 1

The values are means ± standard error of the mean in 4 animals.

Discussion

The first point we shall stress is the physiological state of the mice during the [^{14}C]-DG experiment. Whereas the mice subjected to relative restraint had high glycemia values, possibly related to their reactivity to the partial immobilization, those from the second group were apparently in a normal physiological state, judging by their biological variables and their behavior.

Moreover, despite the occlusion of the common carotid artery, there were no obvious differences between the right and left hemispheres, neither in the EEG activity (fig. 3) nor in LCGU. These results were in keeping with those published by *Pulsinelli and Duffy* [5] in control rats submitted to the same surgical procedure.

In the free-moving mice, the LCGU is relatively constant and its pattern similar to that found in the rat, with average values in gray matter structures higher and more heterogeneous than those in white matter. In both species, the most metabolically active structures are those involved in auditory function (inferior colliculi, auditory cortex, superior olives, medial geniculate bodies) with the highest values in the area of the inferior colliculus. Some other structures, which are involved in motor activity (vestibular nuclei, cerebellar nuclei, floculus, vermis), also have a high rate of glucose consumption. A relatively similar pattern has been described in rats submitted to light motor restraint. It is interesting to notice that the differences in LCGU between auditory and motor structures are less important in our mice than in the rat, a variation possibly related to the free-moving behavior [1, 2].

However, the most metabolically active structures in the mouse have lower LCGU values than the corresponding ones in the rat [8]. This difference is more likely due to the utilization of constants derived from the rat than to the activity of our mice since the ratio of LCGU in gray matter to that in white matter is similar to this ratio in the rat [3, 9].

This preliminary work demonstrates the possibility of measuring the rates of energy metabolism in specific brain structures of free-moving mice. It represents a step towards the utilization of this technique in studying the correlations between physiological or pathological behavior and glucose consumption.

Acknowledgments

Special thanks are expressed to Dr. *Jacques Mouret* for stimulating discussions and for help in writing the manuscript, and to Dr. *Pierre Bobillier* for encouraging the initial steps of this study.

References

1 Brodal, A.: Anatomy of vestibular nuclei and their connections; in Handbook of sensory physiology. Part 1. Vestibular system (1974).

2 Chambers, W.W.; Sprague, J.M.: Functional organization in the cerebellum. Organization in longitudinal and cortico-nuclear zones and their contribution to the control of posture, both extrapyramidal and pyramidal. J. comp. Neurol. *103:* 105–129 (1955).

3 Des Rosiers, M.H.; Descarries, L.: Adaptation de la méthode au désoxyglucose à l'échelle cellulaire: préparation histologique du système nerveux central en vue de la radioautographie à haute résolution. C. r. hebd. Séanc. Acad. Sci., Paris *287:* 153–156 (1978).

4 Kennedy, C.; Sakurada, O.; Shinohara, M.; Jehle, J.W.; Sokoloff, L.: Local cerebral glucose utilization in the normal conscious macaque monkey. Ann. Neurol. *4:* 293–301 (1978).

5 Pulsinelli, W.A.; Duffy, T.E.: Local cerebral metabolism during controlled hypoxemia in rats. Science *204:* 626–629 (1979).

6 Reivich, M.; Jehle, J.W.; Sokoloff, L.; Kety, S.S.: Measurement of regional cerebral blood flow with antipyrine [^{14}C] in awake cats. J. appl. Physiol. *27:* 296–300 (1969).

7 Sidman, R.L.; Green, M.C.; Appel, S.H.: Catalog of the neurological mutants of the mouse, p. 82 (Harvard University Press, Cambridge 1965).

8 Sokoloff, L.; Reivich, M.; Kennedy, C.; Des Rosiers, M.H.; Patlak, C.S.; Pettigrew, K.D.; Sakurada, O.; Shinohara, M.: The [^{14}C] deoxyglucose method for the measurement of local cerebral glucose utilization: theory, procedure and normal values in the conscious and anesthetized albino rat. J. Neurochem. *28:* 897–916 (1977).

9 Sokoloff, L.: Relation between physiological function and energy metabolism in the central nervous system. J. Neurochem. *29:* 13–26 (1977).

T. Nowaczyk, Inserm U-52, Département de Médecine Expérimentale, Faculté de Médecine, 8, avenue Rockefeller, F-69373 Lyon Cédex 2 (France)

Eur. Neurol. *20:* 173–175 (1981)

Alterations in Local Glucose Consumption following Systemic Administration of Kainic Acid, Bicuculline or Metrazol

Y. Ben-Ari, D. Riche, E. Tremblay, G. Charton

Laboratoire de Physiologie nerveuse, Département de Neurophysiologie appliquée, CNRS, Gif-sur-Yvette, France

Key Words. Epilepsy · Deoxyglucose · Kainic acid · Bicuculline · Metrazol · Brain pathology

Abstract. Using the autoradiographic deoxyglucose method, local consumption of glucose has been visualized during convulsive seizures induced by systemic administration of kainic acid, bicuculline or metrazol. A striking correlation was found between the time course of the electrographic and metabolic alterations in limbic structures following kainic acid administration. In addition, pathological alterations were almost exclusively observed in structures in which there had been a rise in metabolism. In contrast, following bicuculline or metrazol a rise in metabolism was conspicuous primarily in the cerebellum, vestibular nuclei and neocortex.

Introduction

Limbic structures are notorious for their vulnerability to the pathological sequelae of the epilepsies. Thus, the presence of pathological alterations in the hippocampal formation of patients having suffered from epilepsies is well documented [4]. The reasons for this vulnerability to epilepsy is poorly understood. Evidence derived from experiments utilizing systemic administration of the convulsant alkaloid bicuculline suggests that the hippocampal sclerosis cannot be readily attributable to known systemic consequences of the seizures [6]. More recently utilizing intra-amygdaloid injections of kainic acid (KA) – a model which reproduces a similar pattern of brain vulnerability [2] – several observations were made which strongly suggest that local factors closely related to the seizure discharge per see may be of particular importance for formation of the hippocampal lesions [3]. If paroxysmal discharge can produce pathological alterations in limbic structures, it is essential to investigate the local metabolic changes which occur during enhanced neuronal discharge in order to gain a better understanding of the relationship between epilepsy and brain pathology. The 2-deoxyglucose method [2-DG – see ref. 8] has been utilized for this purpose in the present study.

Material and Methods

In brief [1], male Wistar rats (250–300 g) received a single injection of KA (9 mg/kg i.p.) and the electrographic and clinical signs were noted. Following various delays (10 min to 3 days) a pulse of 2-deoxy-*D*-(^{14}C) glucose (CEA, specific activity 40–50 uCi/μ*M*) was injected in the jugular vein, in the unanesthetized, unrestrained animal, through a chronically implanted catheter. After a delay of 45 min the brain was rapidly removed and processed for conventional autoradiography (16 μm thickness frontal or sagittal sections, Mammuray T3 films, 3 weeks' exposure). In additional experiments, the animals received a 2-DG pulse followed 3 min later by a single injection of bicuculline (0.9 mg/kg, i.v.) or metrazol (60 mg/kg, i.p.). The brains were similarly treated for autoradiography. Pathological alterations were investigated by means of the Fink-Heimer, Klüver and Barrera or Nissl stains using the unfixed 2-DG labelled sections or from conventionally prepared fixed material obtained in a separate experimental series.

Results

As described in detail elsewhere [3] systemic administration of KA induces typical limbic seizures. Clinically, the animals display wet shakes, paw tremor, head noddings, mastication and rearing on the hind paws as well as an abundant salivation. Electrographically, paroxysmal discharge is noted first (20 min after the injection) exclusively in the hippocampal formation (in particular the entorhinal cortex and Ammon's horn); the epileptiform activity involves at longer delays other 'limbic' structures (amygdala, medial thalamus, prefrontal cortex). The first typical limbic motor seizure is noted approximately 1 h after the injection. At longer delays (2–3 days) epileptiform activity is exclusively seen in the amygdaloid complex. Short delays after the injection (i.e. less than 1 h, when the animal had not displayed full limbic motor seizures) an increased glucose consumption is exclusively seen in the hippocampal formation. 2–4 h after the injection (when the animal had displayed several recurrent limbic motor seizures and often status epilepticus) the increase in radioactive material is seen to involve structures which are part of or closely associated to the limbic system, and in addition to the hippocampal formation, the lateral septum and the fornix system, the claustrum, prefrontal and cingulate cortices, mediodorsal and adjacent medial thalamic nuclei, the amygdala and bed nucleus of the stria terminalis, ventral striatum and various parts of the olfactory system. Concomitantly, a considerable decrease in glucose consumption is seen in most remaining structures of the brain. At longer delays (2–3 days), a considerable decrease is manifest in the entire brain with the noticeable exception of the amygdaloid complex (thus in keeping with the electrographic data). Pathological alterations are almost exclusively noted in structures in which there had been a rise in metabolism (in particular the hippocampal formation, lateral septum, amygdala, claustrum and medial thalamus).

In contrast, bicuculline or metrazol produce less than 1 min after the injection a typical tonico-clonic generalized convulsive seizure involving the entire neocortical mantle. After short delays after one or a few generalized convulsive seizures, the most conspicuous rise in metabolism is noted in the cerebellum and vestibular nuclei, the red nucleus, substantia nigra, nucleus of the oculomotor never and neocortex. A decrease was often manifest in limbic structures (including the amygdala and hippocampal formation). After short delays the most conspicuous brain damage noted with the Fink-Heimer stain is seen in the cerebellar cortex.

Therefore, in our experimental conditions [7] the scattered pathological alterations seen in limbic structures do not appear to correlate to a previous enhancement of neuronal metabolism.

Discussion

The results summarized in the present report confirm the exceptional usefulness of the deoxyglucose method for the study of the relationship between epilepsy and brain pathology. In addition, the possibility of preparing the brains without affecting the radioactive material [5] should permit comparison on the same sections the distribution of labelled material at the cellular level and the pathological alterations.

The observations obtained with KA clearly suggest that in limbic structures, in particular in Ammon's horn, an increase of the neuronal discharge and metabolism is associated with characteristic pathological alterations. In addition there is a remarkable correlation between the time course of electrographic and metabolic alterations. The striking correlation between local metabolic rate and pathological alterations suggest that the development of cell damage is intimately related to the excessive enhancement in neuronal activity and metabolism. In contrast to KA, systemic administration of metrazol or bicuculline readily produced a grand mal tonico-clonic convulsion. In keeping with a large number of previous investigations, both convulsants produced with a swift onset a fully generalized paroxysmal activity with, however, a preferential involvement of neocortical structures. In accordance with the different etiologies, the 2-DG maps were almost negative images of that obtained after KA.

References

1 Ben-Ari, Y.; Riche, D.; Tremblay, E.; Charton, G.: Etat de mal épileptique produit par l'administration systémique d'acide kaïnique: cartographie métabolique à l'aide de la méthode au déoxyglucose. C.r. hebd. Séanc. Acad. Sci., Paris *290:* 1149–1151 (1980).

2 Ben-Ari, Y.; Tremblay, E.; Ottersen, O.P.: Injections of kainic acid into the amygdaloid complex of the rat: an electrographic, clinical and histological study in relation to the pathology of epilepsy. Neuroscience *5:* 515–528 (1980).

3 Ben-Ari, Y.; Tremblay, E.; Ottersen, O.P.; Meldrum, B.S.: The role of epileptic activity in hippocampal and 'remote' cerebral lesions induced by kainic acid. Brain Res. *191:* 79–97 (1980).

4 Blackwood, W.; Corsellis, J.A.N.: Greenfield's neuropathology (Arnold, London 1976).

5 Des Rosiers, M.H.; Descarries, L.: Adaptation de la méthode au déoxyglucose à l'échelle cellulaire: préparation histologique du système nerveux central en vue de la radioautographie à haute résolution . C.r. hebd. Séanc. Acad. Sci., Paris *287:* 153–156 (1978).

6 Meldrum, B.S.; Vigouroux, R.A.; Brierley, J.B.: Systemic factors and epileptic brain damage. Archs Neurol., Chicago *29:* 82–87 (1973).

7 Siesjo, B.K.; Abdul-Rahman, A.: A metabolic basis for the selective vulnerability of neurons in status epilepticus. Acta physiol. scand. *106:* 377–378 (1979).

8 Sokoloff, L.: Mapping of local cerebral functional activity by measurement of local cerebral glucose utilisation with ^{14}C-deoxyglucose. Brain Res. *102:* 653–668 (1980).

Y. Ben-Ari, Laboratoire de Physiologie nerveuse, Département de Neurophysiologie appliquée, CNRS, F–91190 Gif-sur-Yvette (France)

Eur. Neurol. *20:* 176–179 (1981)

Effect of Chloral Hydrate Anaesthesia on the Cerebral Metabolic Response to Apomorphine Administration

J.J. Grome, J. McCulloch

Wellcome Surgical Institute, University of Glasgow, United Kingdom

Key Words. Chloral hydrate · Deoxyglucose · Apomorphine · Cerebral metabolism

Abstract. Using the quantitative ^{14}C-2-deoxyglucose method to measure glucose utilisation in discrete areas of the brain, we have shown that chloral hydrate anaesthesia causes a marked depression of cerebral metabolism in all grey matter areas measured. Moreover, chloral hydrate anaesthesia can reduce, abolish or reverse the action of apomorphine upon glucose utilisation from that seen in conscious animals.

Introduction

The quantitative 2-deoxyglucose method has been used in conscious rats to study functional changes in discrete areas of the brain following manipulation of the central dopaminergic system [3, 4]. In contrast, much of the information previously available concerning the possible role of dopamine in the central nervous system has been based on neurochemical and electrophysiological investigations in anaesthetised animals, with chloral hydrate being particularly widely used [see 1, 2, 6 for examples].

The present study had two aims: (1) to investigate the effect of chloral hydrate anaesthesia on local cerebral glucose utilisation, and (2) to study the effect of chloral hydrate on the response of discrete areas of the brain to the putative dopaminergic agonist, apomorphine.

Methods

The experiments were carried out on 16 male Sprague-Dawley rats (320–400 g). Catheters were implanted in the femoral artery and vein under light halothane anaesthesia.

Conscious Animals. After surgery, these animals were prepared as described in detail by *Sokoloff* et al. [5], and allowed to recover for 2 h before apomorphine administration.

Anaesthetised Animals. After the animals were tracheotomised and catheterised, chloral hydrate was administered (100 mg/kg, i.v., maintained subsequently by a constant infusion of 3 mg/kg/min), the gaseous anaesthetic was withdrawn and the animal was subsequently ventilated with room air for at least 30 min before apomorphine was administered (1 mg/kg, i.v.).

Measurement of Glucose Utilisation. Apomorphine dissolved in saline, or vehicle alone, was administered 10 min before 50 μCi of ^{14}C-2-deoxyglucose was injected intravenously as a bolus. The measurement of glucose utilisation was then carried out, using the quantitative autoradiographic method as described in full by *Sokoloff* et al. [5].

Results

Local glucose utilisation was measured in 30 discrete areas of the brain in both conscious and anaesthetised groups. Data are presented as mean ± standard error of the means.

Effects of Chloral Hydrate Anaesthesia

Glucose utilisation decreased markedly in all grey matter areas measured in the anaesthetised control group when compared to the conscious controls. There was a variation in this depression of 12–52% from structure to structure. Cortical and thalamic structures tended to be more affected than limbic areas (e.g. hippocampus) and some extrapyramidal structures (e.g. substantia nigra) (table I).

Attenuation of Response. A number of structures showed a significant response in both conscious and anaesthetised animals, although in each case the response to apomorphine administration was severely attenuated by chloral hydrate anaesthesia; for example, globus pallidus and subthalamic nucleus (table II).

Table I. Local glucose utilisation (μmol/100 g/min)

Structures	Conscious controls	Anaesthetised controls
Cerebral cortex		
Auditory	127 ± 8	62 ± 5***
Parietal	86 ± 4	49 ± 3***
Sensorimotor	93 ± 4	52 ± 3***
Anterior cingulate	87 ± 7	57 ± 3*
Extrapyramidal and sensorimotor areas		
Thalamus (mediodorsal)	87 ± 4	52 ± 7***
Thalamus (ventrolateral)	72 ± 3	41 ± 4***
Caudate nucleus	82 ± 2	55 ± 4**
Globus pallidus	48 ± 1	31 ± 2***
Substantia nigra (pars compacta)	65 ± 4	48 ± 2**
Substantia nigra (pars reticulata)	47 ± 4	35 ± 2*
Red nucleus	61 ± 5	38 ± 4**
Limbic areas		
Hippocampus	73 ± 6	58 ± 5*
Dentate gyrus	58 ± 4	45 ± 3*
Nucleus accumbens	68 ± 1	52 ± 5*
Amygdala	41 ± 1	32 ± 2**
White matter tracts		
Corpus callosum	33 ± 3	29 ± 6
Internal capsule	31 ± 3	25 ± 4*

All results expressed as mean ± SEM. For preparation of controls see 'Methods'.
* = $p < 0.05$; ** = $p < 0.01$; *** = $p < 0.001$.

Table II. Local glucose utilisation (μmol/100 g/min)

Response to apomorphine structure	Conscious control	Conscious + apomorphine	Anaesthetised control	Anaesthetised + apomorphine
Attenuation				
Globus pallidus	48 ± 1	71 ± 1***	31 ± 2	40 ± 3*
Subthalamic nucleus	70 ± 1	124 ± 4***	44 ± 1	53 ± 3*
Blockade				
Sensorimotor cortex	93 ± 4	158 ± 11**	52 ± 3	56 ± 3
Red nucleus	65 ± 5	89 ± 3**	38 ± 4	42 ± 4
Reversal				
Substantia nigra (pars compacta)	65 ± 4	80 ± 1*	48 ± 2	37 ± 2*

All results expressed as mean ± SEM. For description of animal preparation and apomorphine administration, see 'Methods'.
* = $p < 0.05$; ** = $p < 0.01$; *** = $p < 0.001$.

Blockade or Response. A number of structures which showed significant changes in the conscious group after apomorphine administration produced no significant response in the anaesthetised group; for example, the sensorimotor cortex and the red nucleus (table II).

Reversal of Response. The most important observation made in this study is reversal of the response of the substantia nigra (pars compacta) to apomorphine administration caused by chloral hydrate anaesthesia (table II).

No Change in Glucose Utilisation. Alterations in the rate of glucose utilisation were highly restricted in their distribution in conscious animals, with the majority of regions examined showing no significant change. Moreover, in anaesthetised animals apomorphine failed to alter the glucose utilisation in these areas.

Discussion

As one might logically expect, these data show that chloral hydrate anaesthesia markedly depresses local glucose utilisation in grey matter areas; white matter areas being affected to a lesser extent. Cerebral glucose utilisation thus tends to become more homogeneous throughout the central nervous system. Furthermore, there is a tendency for areas associated with sensory function to be more affected by anaesthesia than limbic areas (table I). These results are in general agreement with previously published data on the consequences of barbiturate and γ-butyrolactone anaesthesia on cerebral glucose utilisation as compared to conscious controls [5, 7].

In this study, we have presented information on the effects of chloral hydrate anaesthesia changes in glucose utilisation following apomorphine administration. Chloral hydrate anaesthesia results in quantitative and qualitative alterations in the pattern of metabolic responses to apomorphine administration. This anaesthetic regime can block (e.g. sensorimotor cortex) or attenuate (e.g. subthalamic nucleus) the action of apomorphine on cerebral glucose utilisation (table II). Chloral hydrate anaesthesia alters not only the normal pattern of glucose utilisation, but also alters the response of the central nervous system to apomorphine administration. It is our view, however, that the most important result of the present investigation concerns the action of apomorphine on the substantia nigra (pars compacta). Dopamine-containing cell bodies within this structure provide the major dopaminergic innervation of forebrain structures.

A number of investigators have shown that apomorphine administration causes a marked depression in the firing rate of these dopamine cell bodies. In many instances, these investigations were carried out on chloral hydrate anaesthetised preparations [1, 6, for examples]. Our results, in which a similar anaesthetic regime was used, compare favourably, in a qualitative manner, with their results. However, since apomorphine administration in the conscious group produced an opposite response, caution is suggested in the interpretation of data obtained using chloral hydrate anaesthetised preparations, particularly in the case of studies of the functional role of the dopaminergic system.

References

1 Bunney, B.S.; Walter, J.R.; Roth, R.H.; Aghajanian, G.K.: Dopaminergic neurons: effects of antipsychotic drugs and amphetamine on single cell activity. J. Pharmac. exp. Ther. *185:* 560–571 (1973).

2 Bunney, B.S.; Aghajanian, G.K.: Dopamine and norepinephrine innervated cells in the rat prefrontal cortex. Life Sci. *19:* 1783–1792 (1976).

3 McCulloch, J.; Savaki, H.E.; McCulloch, M.C.; Sokoloff, L.: Specific distribution of metabolic alterations in cerebral cortex following apomorphine administration. Nature, Lond. *282:* 303–305 (1979).

4 McCulloch, J.; Savaki, H.E.; Sokoloff, L.: Influence of dopaminergic systems on the lateral habenular nucleus of the rat. Brain Res. *194:* 117–124 (1980).

5 Sokoloff, L.; Reivich, M.; Kennedy, C.; Des Rosiers, M.H.; Patlak, C.S.; Pettigrew, K.D.; Sakurada, O.; Shinohara, M.: The ^{14}C-deoxyglucose method for the measurement of local cerebral glucose utilisation. Theory, procedure and normal values in the conscious and anaesthetised albino rat. J. Neurochem. *28:* 897–917 (1977).

6 Van der Heyden, J.A.M.; Venema, K.; Korf, J.: Biphasic and opposite effects of dopamine and apomorphine on endogenous GABA release in the rat substantia nigra. J. Neurochem. *34:* 119–125 (1980).

7 Wolfson, L.I.; Sakurada, O.; Sokoloff, L.: Effects of γ-butyrolactone on local cerebral glucose utilisation in the rat. J. Neurochem. *29:* 777–783 (1977).

J.J. Grome, Wellcome Surgical Institute, University of Glasgow, Glasgow (United Kingdom)

Eur. Neurol. *20:* 180–182 (1981)

Specific Behavior-Bound Brain Cartography of the Glucose Uptake Rate

S. Nicolaidis[a], *M. Le Poncin-Lafitte*[b], *J. Danguir*[a], *C. Grosdemouge*[b], *J.R. Rapin*[b]

[a]CNRS-Collège de France et [b]Neurophysiologie cérébrovasculaire, CHU St-Antoine, Paris, France

Key Words. Deoxyglucose uptake · Dehydration · Thirst

Abstract. The 2-deoxyglucose uptake method studied by autoradiography was used to determine the modification produced by a thirst-dependent state. The density of the subfornical organ, the suprachiasmatic area and the nucleus medianus was higher in dehydrated than in normohydrated animals. These areas are certainly involved in the detection of dehydration and in thirst.

Introduction

The rate of glucose utilization revealed by labelled 2-deoxy-*D*-glucose (2-DG), as described by *Sokoloff* et al. [7], can be a useful tool in determining the brain locations involved in a number of specific functions. This methodology may be impossible to apply in investigations of physiological states linked to behavioral responses because of the 45-min interval between the 2-DG injection and the sacrifice. An alternative method was proposed [4] measuring the 2-DG uptake only 3 min after this injection. This technique enables better investigations of dynamic changes of both physiological states and behavior. We propose such an approach illustrated by a paradigm of thirst-dependent states. The data obtained from these investigations can by no means be considered as definitive, particularly because of the small number of subjects.

Their interest resides in the description of the methodology used and also in the possibility of revealing anatomical structures activated by the extracellular and intracellular dehydration underlying the state not only of thirst but also of antidiuresis and of neuroendocrinological changes such as high levels of circulating and cerebral angiotensin II (AII).

Methods

2 control and 2 experimental animals were used in this experiment. Experimental rats were dehydrated by means of water deprivation during 48 h. This deprivation induces a combined intracellular and extracellular dehydration. Food was present for all subjects;

the control subjects could drink ad libitum during the same period. All rats have been previously equipped with an indwelling catheter in their right atrium. The catheter was fixed on the skull following a previously described technique [2]. A minimum delay of 2 days was allowed for postoperative recovery. If the body weight did not return to the control value, an additional delay was given before the experiment was performed.

On the day of experiment, all rats were connected by means of a P10 polyethylene tubing to an injecting system. The catheter was gently pulled from the roof of the cylindric cage. This type of attachment together with a hydraulic swivel [2] allows the animal to move freely and in addition it can receive intravenous injections. The experiments were performed in their home cages at 11.00. Labelled 2-DG was first injected in a bolus and followed 2.30 min later by ^{125}I-labelled iodoantipyrine also injected as a bolus. 30 s later the animals were sacrificed. The brain was quickly removed and frozen into isopentane surrounded by liquid air. This double labelling allows measurements of both glucose uptake rate [4] and the vascular bed [5].

For autoradiographic studies, 30 serial sections were made. The densitometric comparison of dehydrated versus normohydrated brains was visual. Brain slices of paired animals were treated simultaneously in order to avoid differences in artefacts as much as possible. Alternative slices were used for glucose uptake and for vascular bed measurements.

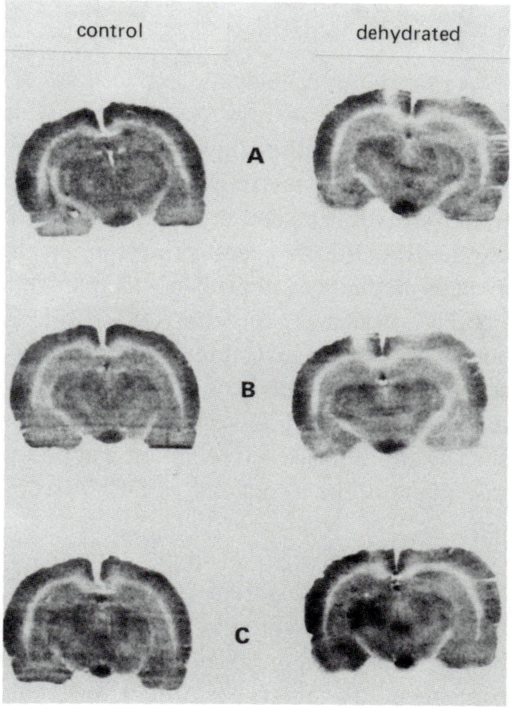

Fig. 1. Autoradiograph of section of conscious rat brain 3 min after deoxyglucose ^{14}C administration (100 µCi). Increase of 2-DG uptake in the brain of the dehydrated rats. A = In the nucleus medianus; B = in the SFO; C = in the suprachiasmatic area.

Results

The visual comparison of the serial sections of the dehydrated and normohydrated brains did not reveal any appreciable difference in 2-DG-induced density in almost all brain areas. However, three regions clearly showed difference of densities. These are the subfornical organ (SFO) area, the zone above the suprachiasmatic area and what seems to be the area of the nucleus medianus (fig. 1). In all of these three areas the density was much higher in dehydrated than in normohydrated animals. Although the extension of labelling seems to be quite restrictive to the SFO and to the nucleus medianus, that of the suprachiasmatic zone certainly includes the organum vasculosum lamina terminalis (OVLT) but it extends towards the preoptic area and to the anterior limits of the median eminence which is not included.

The vascular bed within the same areas was similar in the dehydrated and the normohydrated brains. Although it is difficult to assess, the vascular bed of the dehydrated SFO and OVLT areas seems to be even diminished.

Discussion

A mixed intracellular and extracellular dehydration seems to result in an increase in glucose uptake within three brain structures which have been incriminated in the detection of dehydration and in thirst. These areas are the SFO [6], its neural projection on the nucleus medianus and probably the paraventricular nucleus [1] and the OVLT [3]. In addition the same structures are increasingly suspected to be involved in all of the synergic functions activated in case of dehydration such as antidiuresis, AII secretion and (in the case of extracellular deficits) of DOCA secretion.

The small number of animals makes us cautious in the assessment of specific glucose uptake by the structures which are involved in regulatory responses of dehydration. If confirmed, the observed localization could be interpreted as sustaining the increase rate of glucose utilization by these structures since there was no vascular bed changes susceptible to modify the vascular permeability of hypervascular organs such as the SFO and the OVLT. In addition, the blood-brain barrier is absent at the level of these circumventricular organs. Therefore, the interpretation of difference of densities in terms of change of blood-brain barrier by the dehydrated tissues is unlikely.

References

1 Miselis, R.R.; Hand, P.J.; Berger, R.: An autoradiographic study of the efferent connectivity of the FFO. Proc. VIth Int. Conf. Physiology of Food and Fluid Intake, Paris 1977.

2 Nicolaidis, S.; Rowland, N.; Meile, M.J.; Marfaing-Jallat, P.; Pesez, A.: A flexible technique for long-term infusion in unrestrained rats. Pharmacol. Biochem. Behav. *2:* 131–136 (1974).

3 Nicolaidis, S.; Fitzsimons, J.T.: La dépendance de la prise d'eau induite par l'angiotensine II envers la fonction vasomotrice cérébrale locale chez le rat. C.r. hebd. Séanc. Acad. Sci., Paris *281(D):* 1417–1420 (1975).

4 Rapin, J.R.; Lageron, A.; Le Poncin-Lafitte, M.: Deoxyglucose uptake in pathological conditions. Eur. Neurol. *20:* 146–151 (1981).

5 Rapin, J.R.; Duterte, D.; Le Poncin-Lafitte, M.: Modèles d'étude des désordres cérébrovasculaires à l'aide de déoxyglucose ^{3}H. Radioakt. Isotope Klin. Forsch. *14:* 269–276 (1980).

6 Simpson, J.B.; Routtenberg, A.: Subfornical organ: site of drinking elicitation by angiotensin II. Science *181:* 1172–1175 (1973).

7 Sokoloff, L.; Reivich, M.; Kennedy, C.; Des Rosiers, M.H.; Patlak, C.S.; Pettigrew, K.D.; Sakurada, O.; Shinohara, M.: The ^{14}C-deoxyglucose method for the measurement of local cerebral glucose utilization: theory, procedure and normal values in the conscious and anesthetized rat. J. Neurochem. *28:* 897–916 (1977).

S. Nicolaidis, CNRS-Collège de France,
place Marcelin-Berthelot, F–75005 Paris (France)

Eur. Neurol. *20:* 183–187 (1981)

Various Indices of Brain Metabolism and Activity in a Model of Chronic Neurological Dysfunction: Triethyl Tin Intoxication in the Rat

Y. Legrain, E.T. MacKenzie

Department of Biology, LERS, Synthelabo, Bagneux, France

Key Words. Neurologic deficit · Electrocortical activity · Brain tissue concentration: water, K^+, Na^+ · Focal cerebral blood flow · Local cerebral glucose utilization

Abstract. A number of pathological agents of interest in the therapy of cerebrovascular disease can retard the development of the neurologic deficit induced by triethyl tin. Locomotor activity was decreased at a time when no evidence of neurologic deficit could be detected. Conduction velocity in the peripheral as well as the central nervous system were essentially unmodified. Impairment of brain function as assessed from measurement of cerebral blood flow, local cerebral glucose utilization, brain water and electrolyte content as well as neuropathology were measured before any frank deficit could be clinically detected.

Introduction

The deliberate intoxication of experimental animals with various salts of triethyl tin is known to effect a widespread disturbance of the central nervous system; a peripheral neuropathy is encountered in the more advanced stages of the intoxication [1, 2]. In the central nervous system, the development of brain oedema has been one of the most studied phenomena and it is known that this oedema can be minimized by treatment with corticosteroids [3, 4]. However, at the molecular level, triethyl tin (TET) is known to influence the coupling between oxidative phosphorylation and electron transport, and to inhibit the synthesis of ATP by cerebral mitochondria or cortical slices [5, 6].

A number of pharmacological agents of interest in the therapy of cerebrovascular disease can retard the development of the neurological deficit induced by TET intoxication (fig. 1a). It was with this background that it was thought worthwhile to characterize a number of pathophysiological changes during TET intoxication in the hope that a further understanding would be gained of the mechanism of action of TET in this experimental model.

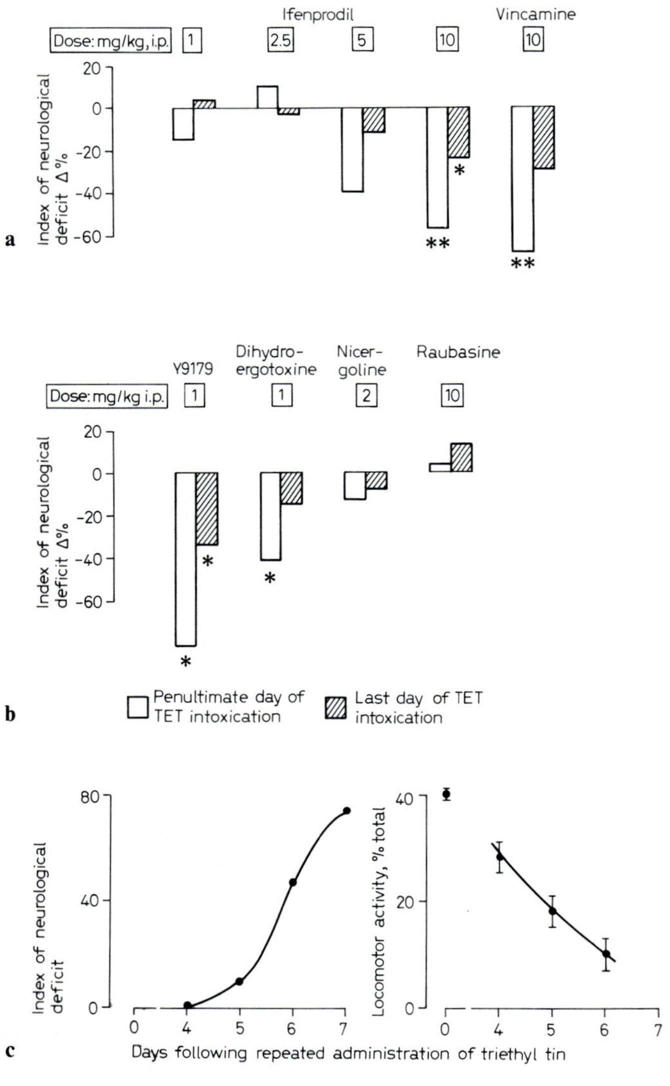

Fig. 1. **a** Illustrative presentation of the percentage difference in the index of neurological deficit between drug-treated and matched saline-treated rats on the last 2 days of TET-induced intoxication. The calculation of this difference is explained in the text. Statistical difference was tested by the Chi square test where * = $p < 0.05$ and ** = $p < 0.01$. **b** Increase of the index of neurological dysfunction (weighed sum of the rating scale of neurological deficit, as defined in the text). **c** Decrease of the overall locomotor activity (expressed as percentage of the total recorded time). Each value is given as mean ± SEM.

Methods and Results

In the present study, TET was given daily by the oral route (2 mg/kg). Some of the experiments were performed in rats lightly anaesthetized with N_2O, curarized and mechanically ventilated so as to keep arterial pressure, blood gas tensions as well as pH in the normal range.

Neurological Investigations

A rating scale was defined to score the neurological deficit where 1 = loss of spontaneous motor activity, 2 = loss of the hind limb grasping reflex, 3 = loss of withdrawal reflexes, moribund and dead. Addition of individual scores for a group of rats was used to define the group neurological deficit index. Essentially no major abnormalities were observed on day 4; the slight deficit rated on day 5 was due to the disappearance of spontaneous locomotor activity in a few rats; then the deficit increased due to animals losing the grasping reflex and in the last day to animals losing the withdrawal reflex or which were dead. An illustrative presentation of the difference, expressed as a percentage, between the neurological deficit index calculated in a group of 15 drug-treated rats and a group of 15 matched saline-treated rats is given (fig. 1b). However, locomotor activity measured over 12 h during the night was significantly decreased on day 4, that is when no obvious clinical abnormalities could be detected. A further decrease was recorded on day 5 and 6 (fig. 1c).

A strong and quick withdrawal reflex was still persistent in those animals indicating that the measured behavioural alterations were not due to an excessive muscular weakness. Furthermore, conduction velocity measured on a peripheral nerve of the tail was essentially unaffected throughout the intoxication (32.9 ± 0.9 m/s in 8 control rats, versus 31.6 ± 0.8 m/s in 11 rats on day 5). In addition, the latency of somatosensory potentials was increased when the potential was evoked by electrical stimulation of the contralateral forepaw as well as by stimulation of the contralateral hind paw (8.7 ± 0.4 ms in 9 control rats versus 12.1 ± 0.7 ms in 11 rats on day 5). However, the difference between latency measured following stimulation of the forepaw and latency measured following stimulation of the hind paw remained constant for each rat. This indicated that, in the present experimental conditions, conduction velocity was not impaired in the peripheral nervous system and in the spinal cord. A central dysfunction must, therefore, be implicated.

Investigations of Brain Function

ECoG recorded on day 5 appeared essentially unmodified. This is supported by data from power spectrum analysis as well as from calculation of Hjorth parameters (activity, mobility, complexity were respectively 25.9 ± 3.6 μV^2, 8.37 ± 0.47 Hz, 17.28 ± 0.42 in 6 control rats versus 31.7 ± 2.2 μV^2, 9.43 ± 0.6 Hz, 17.75 ± 0.34 in 6 rats intoxicated with 5 doses of TET).

Neuropathology performed in perfusion-fixed brains indicated that brain tissue was altered as soon as day 4. Studies performed in a double-blind way indicated that the severity of the alteration progressively increased during the intoxication.

Local cerebral flow, as measured from the ^{14}C-ethanol technique, was significantly reduced on day 5 in all structures studied (table I); a further decrease was measured on day 6 and 7. Local cerebral glucose utilization (LCGU) was measured according to the tech-

Table I. Brain water and electrolyte content, focal cerebral blood flow and local glucose utilization measured on the fifth, sixth and seventh days following repeated administration of TET

	Untreated rats	Following repeated administration of TET		
		5 days	6 days	7 days
Brain water and electrolyte content				
$[H_2O]$, %	$^{9}78.5 \pm 0.1$	$^{11}79.6 \pm 0.2$***	$^{7}80.4 \pm 0.2$***	$^{7}80.8 \pm 0.2$***
$[Na^+]$, mEq/kg	$^{5}54.9 \pm 0.9$	$^{11}61.9 \pm 1.5$**	$^{4}64.1 \pm 0.8$***	$^{5}68.5 \pm 1.4$***
$[K^+]$, mEq/kg	$^{5}107.6 \pm 1.2$	$^{11}103.2 \pm 3.6$	$^{4}92.1 \pm 0.7$***	$^{5}88.8 \pm 2.1$***
Focal cerebral blood flow, ml/100 g · min				
Frontal cortex	$^{9}188 \pm 15$	$^{5}124 \pm 29$*	$^{7}76 \pm 17$***	$^{7}51 \pm 19$***
Parietal cortex	$^{9}172 \pm 12$	$^{5}121 \pm 32$	$^{7}80 \pm 10$***	$^{7}64 \pm 18$***
Occipital cortex	$^{9}128 \pm 9$	$^{5}84 \pm 16$*	$^{7}55 \pm 9$***	$^{7}40 \pm 12$***
Caudate nucleus	$^{9}125 \pm 9$	$^{5}78 \pm 16$*	$^{7}58 \pm 11$***	$^{7}44 \pm 13$***
Thalamus	$^{9}86 \pm 6$	$^{5}75 \pm 14$	$^{7}56 \pm 8$**	$^{7}52 \pm 15$*
Cerebellum	$^{9}66 \pm 3$	$^{5}50 \pm 7$*	$^{7}38 \pm 2$***	$^{7}36 \pm 5$***
Local glucose utilization, μmol/100 g · min				
Frontal cortex	$^{4}67.6 \pm 2.4$	$^{4}49.5 \pm 1.3$***	$^{4}47.8 \pm 6.1$*	$^{2}47.9 \pm 1$**
Parietal cortex	$^{4}62.8 \pm 1.8$	$^{4}47.0 \pm 2.0$**	$^{4}48.8 \pm 3.0$**	$^{2}47.3 \pm 2.1$**
Occipital cortex	$^{4}55.6 \pm 1.4$	$^{4}40.5 \pm 2.3$**	$^{4}40.1 \pm 3.5$**	$^{2}38.2 \pm 4.5$**
Caudate nucleus	$^{4}54.5 \pm 4.5$	$^{4}35.1 \pm 3.5$*	$^{4}35.3 \pm 1.1$**	$^{2}36.9 \pm 4.5$
Thalamus	$^{4}60.4 \pm 2.7$	$^{4}45.5 \pm 1.7$**	$^{4}48.2 \pm 5.0$	$^{2}48.8 \pm 3.2$
Cerebellum	$^{4}39.7 \pm 1.4$	$^{4}26.8 \pm 1.2$***	$^{4}27.2 \pm 1.2$***	$^{2}27.2 \pm 3.0$*

The number of rats studied is indicated by superior figures. Statistical comparison versus untreated rats was tested by the t test where * = $p < 0.05$, ** = $p < 0.01$, *** = $p < 0.001$.

nique described by *Sokoloff* et al. [7]. On day 3, LCGU was significantly reduced when compared to the baseline values, but the heterogeneity which is usually observed between various brain regions was preserved. On days 5 and 6 LCGU would appear to be essentially similar to that measured on day 3 (table I).

Discussion

In the present study, LCGU was calculated with respect to kinetic constants derived from normal rats. However, it is possible that these constants may differ in rats intoxicated by TET and therefore, further studies to verify these constants would be desirable. The fact that no further decrease in LCGU could be measured after day 3 is at variance with the decrease of cerebral blood flow which further progressed between days 5, 6 and 7. However, cerebral oedema, as assessed from measurement of brain water content, of potassium and sodium content, progressed on days 5, 6 and 7 (table I).

It might be assumed that the decrease in cerebral blood flow induced by TET was primarily related to an alteration of energy metabolism and secondarily to the progression of brain oedema. This process might well not be dissimilar to the progressive deficit which follows a decrease in the supply of energy to the brain.

References

1 Gerren, M.A.; Groswald, D.E.; Luttges, M.W.: Triethyl tin toxicity as a model for degenerative disorders. Pharmacol. Biochem. Behav. *5:* 299–307 (1976).

2 Marshall, L.F.; Bruce, D.A.; Graham, D.I.; Langfitt, T.W.; Alterations in behavior, brain electrical activity, cerebral blood flow and intracranial pressure produced by triethyl tin sulfate induced cerebral edema. Stroke *7:* 21–25 (1976).

3 Studer, R.K.; Siegel, B.N.; Morgan, J.; Potchen, E.J.: Dexamethasone therapy of triethyl tin induced cerebral edema. Expl Neurol. *38:* 429–437 (1973).

4 Levine, S.; Torrelio, M.: Cerebral inflammation and edema: a model in rats for testing antiinflammatory drugs. Expl Neurol. *56:* 361–369 (1977).

5 Cremer, J.E.: The action of triethyl tin, triethyl lead, ethyl mercury and other inhibitors on the metabolism of brain and kidney slices in vitro using substrates labelled with ^{14}C. J. Neurochem. *9:* 289–298 (1962).

6 Aldrige, W.N.: The biochemistry of organotin compounds. Trialkyltins and oxidative phosphorylation. Biochem. J. *69:* 367–375 (1958).

7 Sokoloff, L.; Reivich, M.; Kennedy, C.; Des Rosiers, M.H.; Patlack, C.S.; Pettigrew, K.D.; Sakurada, O.; Shinohara, M.: The [^{14}C] deoxyglucose method for the measurement of local cerebral glucose utilization: theory, procedure and normal values in the conscious and anesthetized albino rat. J. Neurochem. *28:* 897–915 (1977).

Y. Legrain, LERS, Synthelabo, 31, avenue Paul-Vaillant-Couturier, F–92220 Bagneux (France)

Eur. Neurol. *20:* 188–193 (1981)

A Double Tracer Autoradiographic Technique for Simultaneous Measurement of Cerebral Blood Flow and Cerebral Metabolism in Rats

G. Mies, I. Niebuhr, K.-A. Hossmann

Max-Planck-Institut für Hirnforschung, Forschungsstelle für Hirnkreislaufforschung, Köln, BRD

Key Words. Rats · Double tracer autoradiography · ^{131}I-iodo-antipyrine · ^{14}C-deoxyglucose · CBF · CMR glucose · Coupling of metabolism

Abstract. Double tracer autoradiographic measurement of cerebral blood flow and glucose consumption was performed in rats using ^{131}I-iodo-antipyrine and ^{14}C-deoxyglucose, respectively. Local coupling of blood flow and metabolism was studied under different types of anesthesia (barbiturate, halothane), following experimental tumor implantation, and during penicillin seizures or spreading depression. Both coupling and uncoupling of flow and metabolism was observed in the same tissue section, indicating a considerable degree of variability in local coupling mechanisms.

Introduction

Since the description of a relationship between EEG frequency and cerebral blood flow by *Obrist* et al. [5] and *Ingvar* et al. [1], much attention has been directed to coupling mechanisms in the brain [2]. Most of the earlier experimental work was concerned with the correlation of global flow, global metabolism and global function, but with the introduction of autoradiographic techniques regional and even local coupling processes have become of greater interest.

The conventional autoradiographic techniques allow the investigation of coupling processes between two phenomena: function on one hand, and either blood flow or cerebral metabolism on the other. Local coupling of all three parameters can be investigated only by the use of double tracer tomographic or autoradiographic techniques because this is the only way to assess local flow, local metabolism and function in the same subject.

Recently, *Jones* et al. [3] described a double tracer autoradiographic method using ^{14}C-deoxyglucose and ^{123}I-iodo-antipyrine. ^{123}I has a very short half-life, and it is possible to differentiate between the two isotopes by exposing the same tissue section twice and subtracting the two autoradiograms from each other.

We have modified this technique by choosing ^{131}I-iodo-antipyrine as the short-lived isotope and by adjusting the concentrations of the two isotopes in such a way that blackening of the film during the two exposures is almost exclusively by one isotope only. This avoids the need of subtraction and allows the processing of each film as single tracer autoradiograms [4]. In the following, this technique is used for the study of coupling mechanisms under various physiological and pathophysiological conditions.

Material and Methods

Experimental Procedure

Autoradiographic double tracer experiments were performed in 32 BD IX rats of both sexes. Glucose utilization was measured with ^{14}C-deoxyglucose, and blood flow with ^{131}I-iodo-antipyrine. First, 30 µCi of ^{14}C-deoxyglucose was given intravenously as a bolus, and 30 min later 70–80 µCi ^{131}I-iodo-antipyrine was infused intravenously over a period of 1 min. Blood sampling, removal of the brain and autoradiographic procedures were performed according to the descriptions of *Sokoloff* et al. [7] and *Sakurada* et al. [6]. Brain sections were exposed twice: immediately after the experiment for assaying ^{131}I-iodo-antipyrine, and 8 weeks later – after decay of ^{131}I – for assessment of ^{14}C-deoxyglucose, as has been described before [4]. Cross-contamination of the two tracers was negligible and the two autoradiograms could be processed qualitatively or quantitatively in the same way as single tracer autoradiograms.

Experimental Groups

Four groups of animals were used.

Anesthetic Effects. Rats were anesthetized either with 0.8 halothane or with pentobarbital (50 mg/kg), immobilized and maintained under artificial ventilation throughout the experiment.

Experimental Brain Tumors. Intracerebral tumors were produced by implantation of a rat glioma clone (RGI 2.2, courtesy Dr. *Mennel*) into the right hemisphere.

Focal Penicillin Seizures. 20 µl of sodium penicillin G were applied to the cortical surface. Penicillin was replenished every 10 min until the end of the experiment. Seizure activity was ascertained by recording EEG spike activity (fig. 1).

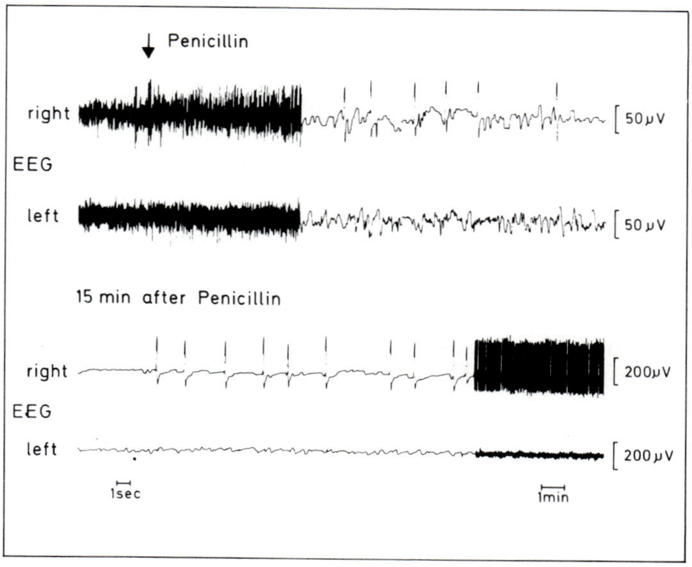

Fig. 1. Recording of seizure activity following topical application of penicillin on the right hemisphere of rat brain.

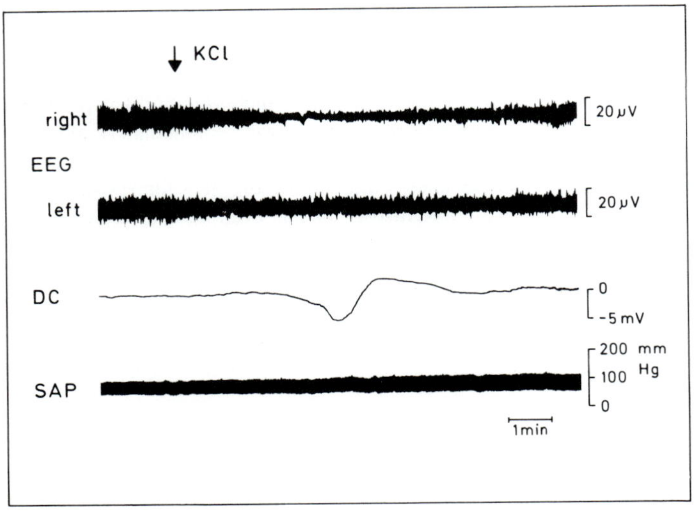

Fig. 2. Recording of EEG, cortical steady potential (DC) and arterial blood pressure (SAP) following topical application of KCl on the right hemisphere of the rat brain.

Spreading Depression. Filter paper soaked with 4 *M* potassium chloride was placed on the exposed dura. Two microcalomel electrodes were positioned over the left and right side of the frontal brain for recording the DC potentials. Successful maintenance of spreading depression was ascertained by suppression of EEG activity and the negative shift of the DC potential, as monitored on a polygraph (fig. 2).

Results and Discussion

Validation of the Method

Details of the autoradiographic double tracer method are described elsewhere [4]. The tissue concentration of ^{131}I being about 50% higher than that of ^{14}C, the latter can be neglected because it contributes to less than 10% of film exposure. The absence of a greater degree of cross-contamination was ascertained in each experiment using appropriate standards.

Animal Experiments

Anesthesia Effects. In rats anesthetized with barbiturate, distribution of flow and metabolism was homogeneous and tightly coupled in all regions of the brain. Under halothane anesthesia a distinct local dissociation between flow and metabolism was present, particularly in the stratum pyramidale of the dorsal hippocampus and the nucleus parafascicularis where an increase in metabolism was not followed by a parallel increase in flow (fig. 3).

Experimental Brain Tumor. In figure 4, the same brain section was assessed for histology, cerebral blood flow and CMR glucose. At higher magnification, it became apparent that within the tumor mass regions of coupled and uncoupled activation of glucose metabolism were present (fig. 4).

Fig. 3. Double tracer autoradiographic demonstration of blood flow and glucose metabolism in rats anesthetized with barbiturate and halothane, respectively.

Fig. 4. Double tracer autoradiography of experimental brain tumor. Below: infiltration zone of tumor at higher magnification.

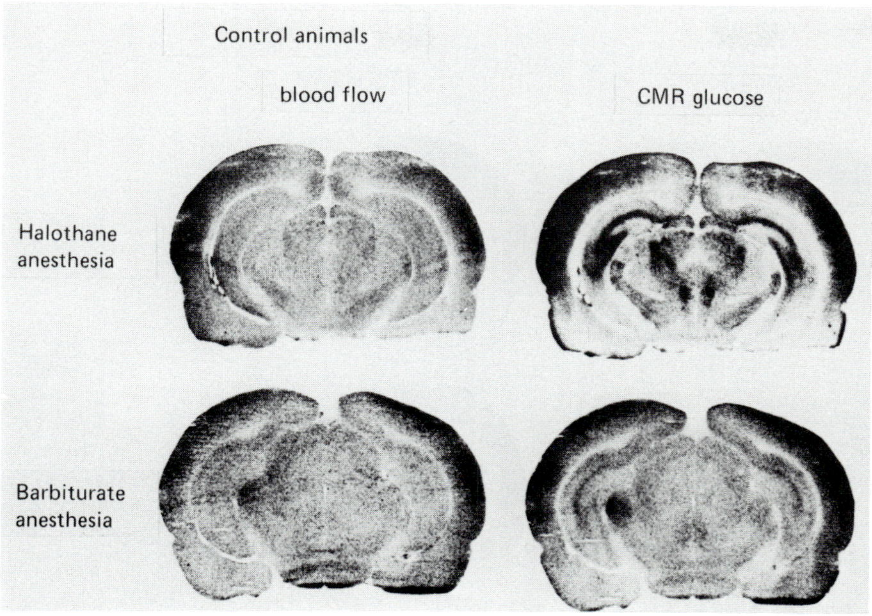
Control animals
blood flow
CMR glucose
Halothane anesthesia
Barbiturate anesthesia

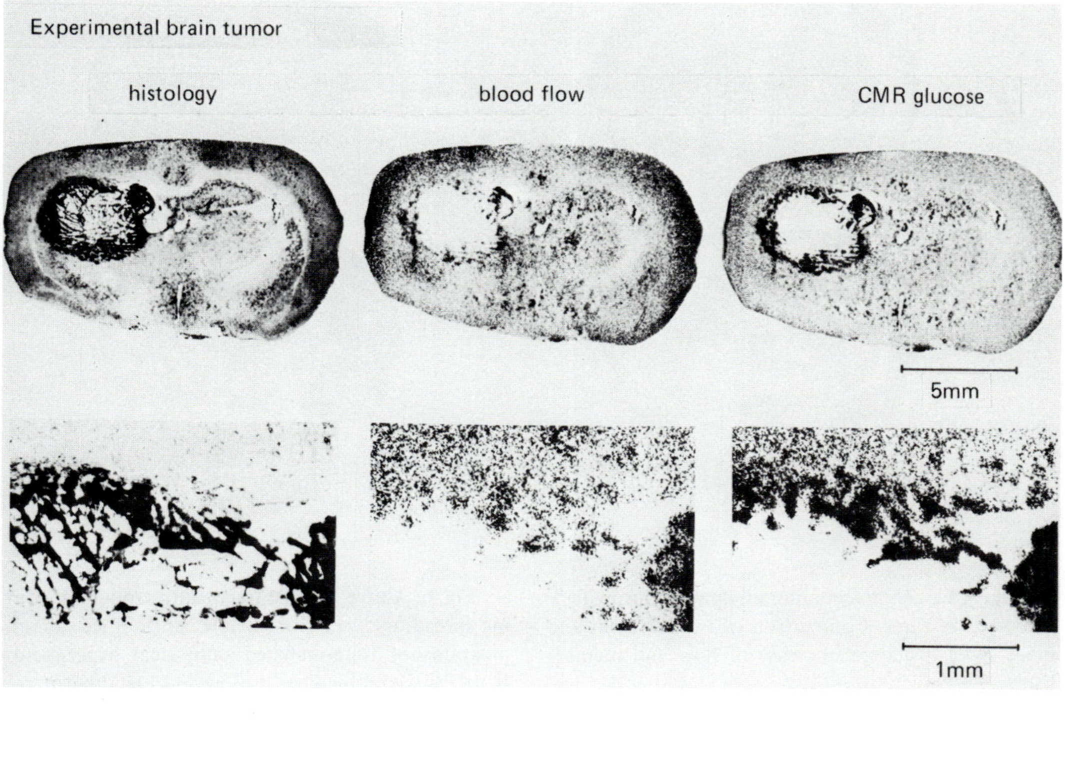
Experimental brain tumor
histology
blood flow
CMR glucose
5mm
1mm

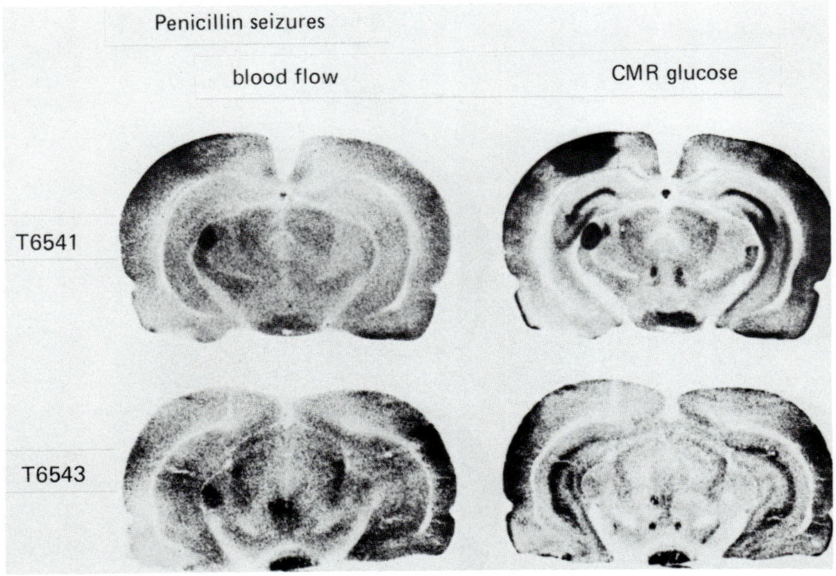

5

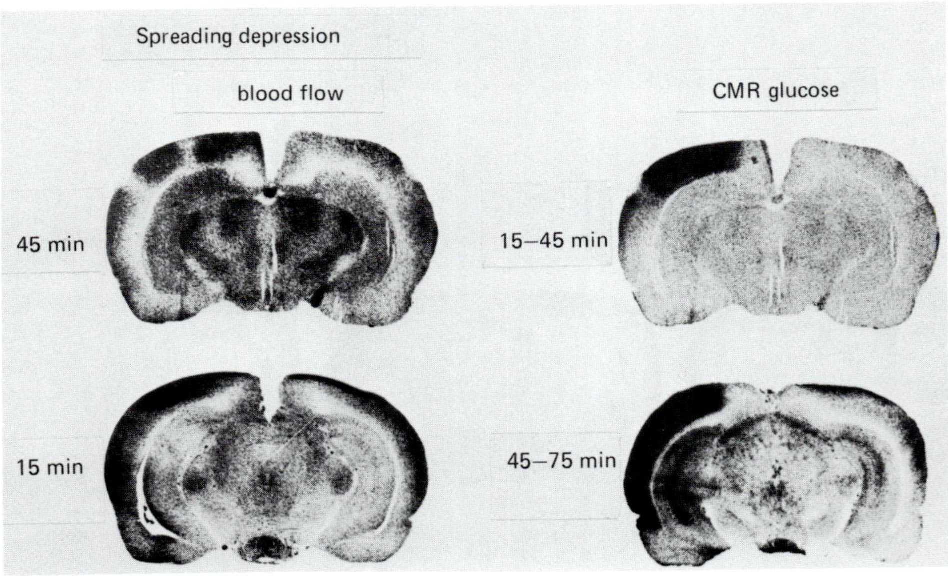

6

Fig. 5. Double tracer autoradiography during focal penicillin seizures. Comparison of two different animals. Note ipsilateral increase of flow and metabolism.

Fig. 6. Above: double tracer autoradiography during spreading depression. Below: single tracer autoradiograms of time-matched individual experiments. Note ipsilateral increase of flow and metabolism.

Penicillin Seizures. In one animal a striking increase in local glucose utilization was observed in the region of penicillin application and in the ipsilateral geniculate body. The increase was coupled to an increase in flow in the thalamic nucleus but not at the site of application. In another animal an increase of flow in the geniculate body without an appropriate increase in glucose utilization could be detected (fig. 5).

Spreading Depression. Glucose utilization was increased at the site of potassium chloride application, and spread over the region supplied by the middle cerebral artery. There was a sharp demarcation against the territory of the anterior cerebral artery in which metabolism was not increased. The associated change in blood flow was much less sharply demarcated against the anterior cerebral artery territory, indicating a certain degree of luxury perfusion at the border of the involved territory. Time-matched single tracer autoradiograms supported the double tracer autoradiographic finding (fig. 6).

The present series of experiments suggests that local coupling of flow and metabolism is not as strict as has been suggested in various reports before [2]. Double tracer autoradiography, therefore, is a necessary tool for the precise local correlation of the two parameters and a prerequisite for studying the involved mechanism at the histological level.

A limitation of the method is the time lag between the application of the two tracers. A precise correlation, therefore, is possible only under steady state conditions during this interval. However, steady state is also a precondition for the accurate application of the deoxyglucose method alone, and the double tracer technique, therefore, can be used in any experimental situation in which this condition is fulfilled.

References

1 Ingvar, D.H.; Baldy-Moulinier, M.; Sulg, I.; Hörman, S.: Regional cerebral blood flow related to EEG. Acta neurol. scand. *14:* suppl., pp. 179–182 (1965).

2 Ingvar, D.H.; Lassen, N.A.: Brain work: the coupling of function, metabolism and blood flow in the brain (Munksgaard, Copenhagen 1975).

3 Jones, S.C.; Lear, J.L.; Greenberg, J.H.; Reivich, M.: A double tracer autoradiographic technique for the quantitative measure of cerebral blood flow and glucose metabolism. Acta neurol. scand. *60:* suppl. 72, pp. 202–203 (1979).

4 Mies, G.; Niebuhr, I.; Hossmann, K.-A.: A new method for simultaneous measurement of blood flow and glucose metabolism by autoradiographic techniques (in preparation).

5 Obrist, W.D.; Sokoloff, L.; Lassen, N.A.; Lane, M.H.; Butler, R.N.; Feinberg, I.: Relation of EEG to cerebral blood flow and metabolism in old age. Electroenceph. clin. Neurophysiol. *15:* 610–619 (1963).

6 Sakurada, O.; Kennedy, C.; Jehle, J.; Brown, J.D.; Garbin, G.L.; Sokoloff, L.: Measurement of local cerebral blood flow with iodo-^{14}C-antipyrine. Am. J. Physiol. H *234:* 59–66 (1978).

7 Sokoloff, L.; Reivich, M.; Kennedy, C.; Des Rosiers, M.H.; Patlak, C.S.; Pettigrew, K.D.; Sakurada, O.; Shinohara, M.: The 2-^{14}C-deoxyglucose method for the measurement of local cerebral glucose utilization: theory, procedure and normal values in the conscious and anesthetized albino rat. J. Neurochem. *28:* 897–917 (1977).

G. Mies, Max-Planck-Institut für Hirnforschung, Forschungsstelle für Hirnkreislaufforschung, Ostmerheimerstrasse 200, D-5000 Köln 91 (FRG)

Eur. Neurol. *20:* 194–199 (1981)

Measurements of Cerebral Oxygen Consumption: Advantages and Limitations

Bo K. Siesjö

Laboratory of Experimental Brain Research, University Hospital, Lund, Sweden

Key Words. Brain · Oxygen consumption · Glucose consumption

Abstract. The main methods for measuring oxygen consumption in the brain are briefly discussed and their main advantages and limitations are mentioned. It is concluded that such methods are superior for measuring the metabolic rate in the brain in non-steady-state situations, as well as in conditions leading to a mismatch between oxygen consumption and glucose utilization.

Introduction

Only a few years ago, measurements of cerebral oxygen consumption (CMR_{O_2}) represented virtually the only accurate way of assessing the metabolic rate in the brain. In measuring CMR_{O_2}, most workers have used the *Kety and Schmidt* [1948] inert gas technique, modifications therefore, or techniques that have been validated against it. About 10 years ago, a technique based on another principle was developed in *Ter-Pogossian's* laboratory, one which utilizes ^{15}O as the diffusible tracer [*Ter-Pogossian* et al., 1970; *Raichle* et al., 1976]. By virtue of its capacity to measure *regional* CMR_{O_2} that technique has even larger resources. However, since it requires sophisticated and expensive equipment it has not yet achieved the practical importance of the *Kety and Schmidt* technique.

The newly developed ^{14}C-deoxyglucose technique of *Sokoloff* et al. [1977] allows measurements of *local* glucose consumption (CMR_{gl}) in experimental animals with a resolution of less than 0.5 mm^2. It therefore must be asked whether CMR_{O_2} measurements continue to be useful. As the following discussion will show, such measurements still have their place. Since the issue has been discussed in some detail in recent reviews [*Siesjö,* 1978; *Siesjö* et al., 1980] the present communication only summarizes the main points. We will start by describing the classic *Kety and Schmidt* technique, emphasizing its advantages and disadvantages, and consider some situations in which measurements of CMR_{O_2} give information not easily gained by methods devised to measure glucose utilization.

The Kety and Schmidt techniques

Theory

One of the virtues of this technique is that it is based on a quantitative principle, the law of conservation of matter. Thus, if an inert substance (Q) is introduced into the arterial circulation, the law states that the difference between the amount carried to the brain by the arterial circulation and that leaving by the venous outflow represents what has been taken up by the tissue. For any instant, one can write

$$\frac{dQ_i}{dt} F(C_a - C_{\bar{v}}) \qquad (1)$$

where Q_i is the amount taken up, F is blood flow, and C_a and $C_{\bar{v}}$ are the arterial and mean venous concentrations. If F is constant the equation can be integrated. Furthermore, if diffusion equilibrium is reached between tissue and venous blood we can write

$$CBF = \frac{\pi \cdot C_{\bar{v}}(T)}{\int_0^T (C_a - C_{\bar{v}})dt} \qquad (2)$$

i.e. we obtain CBF as a function of the venous concentration at 'saturation' (time T), the partition coefficient (π), and the integral of the arteriovenous concentration difference during time T.

Procedure and Applications

Kety and Schmidt [1948] used N_2O as the diffusible tracer and measured its arterial and venous concentrations during a 10-min inhalation period. Many subsequent investigators have used radioactive tracers instead (^{85}Krypton, ^{133}Xenon) and analyzed blood concentrations either during saturation [e.g. *Lassen and Munck,* 1955; *Alexander* et al., 1964] or desaturation [*McHenry,* 1963]. The method has also been adopted for experimental animals. This application has also allowed sampling of cerebral venous blood from the superior sagittal sinus, probably yielding values mainly representing *cortical* CBF and CMR_{O_2} [*Homburger* et al., 1946; *Michenfelder* et al., 1968; *Norberg and Siesjö,* 1976].

Potential Errors

The most important potential errors of the technique is the presence of slowly perfused tissue masses, and contamination of venous blood sampled from extracerebral sources. Both errors will lead to a lingering arteriovenous difference in tracer concentration at the end of the saturation (or desaturation) period. The problems encountered can be exemplified by results obtained in rats with sampling of venous blood from the retroglenoid vein [*Nilsson and Siesjö,* 1976]. Figure 1a shows that a relatively marked arteriovenous difference in ^{133}Xenon activity was observed after 10 min of desaturation. This difference is similar to that observed in man [see *Kety and Schmidt,* 1948]. Since measurements of tissue activities in rats showed that desaturation had occurred already before 10 min, the lingering A-V difference must have been due to admixture of extracerebral blood derived from tissues with low blood flow rates. The error could be avoided by clamping the contralateral retroglenoid vein, a procedure that increased flow through the sampling catheter (fig. 1b).

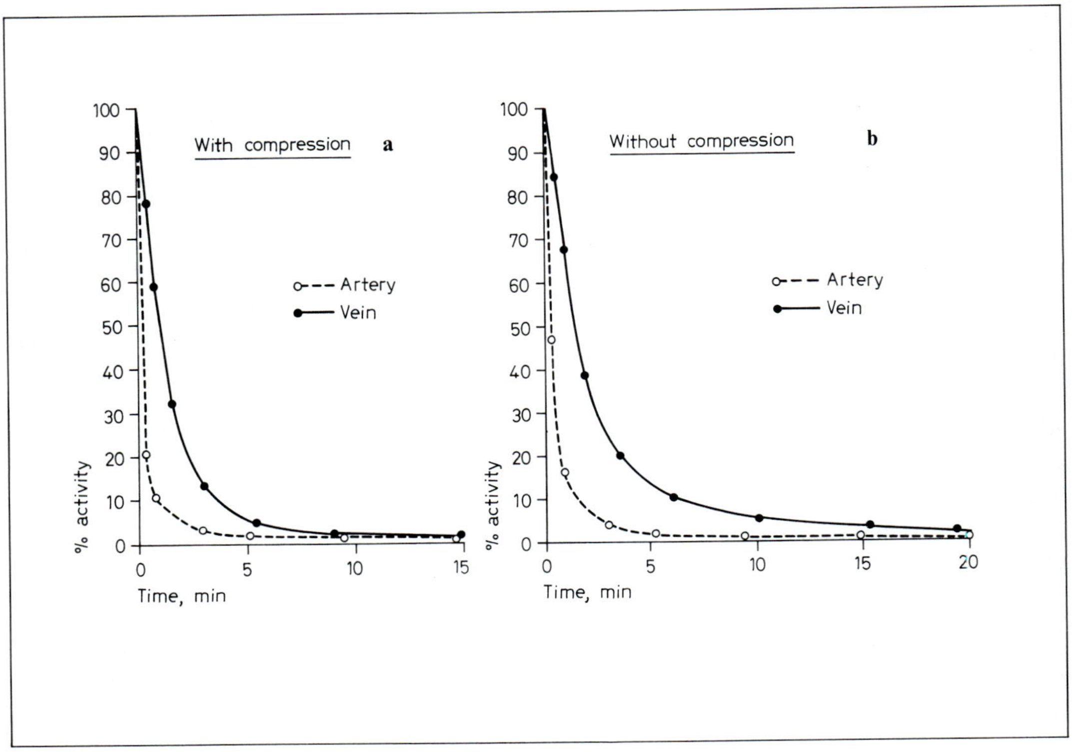

Fig. 1. ^{133}Xe desaturation curves in the rat, using the retroglenoid vein for venous sampling. **a** Curves obtained with compression of contralateral retroglenoid vein during sampling. **b** Typical curves obtained without such compression [from *Nilsson and Siesjö,* 1976].

The errors discussed represent a problem when measuring CBF and CMR_{O_2} in man. Some workers have assumed that a lingering A-V difference after 10 min of saturation/desaturation is due to the presence of slowly perfused masses (e.g. white matter). Accordingly, they have attempted to correct for this by continuing sampling for longer periods, and by extrapolating the A-V differences to infinity [*Lassen and Munck,* 1955; *Lassen and Klee,* 1965; *Alexander* et al., 1964]. However, it should be emphasized that this procedure is inadequate if the cause of the delay in 'equilibration' is due to extracerebral contamination of venous blood.

Validation

At least in the rat, the errors discussed seem to prevent no problems if blood is sampled from the superior sagittal sinus [see *Norberg and Siesjö,* 1976]. In that species, the CBF and CMR_{O_2} data obtained have also been validated by comparison with results derived with other techniques. For example, similar CBF values were obtained by autoradiographic measurements of local blood flow with ^{14}C-iodoantipyrine, and similar results for metabolic rate have been obtained with a kinetic ^{14}C-glucose technique [see *Siesjö* et al., 1980]. Recently, we [*Ingvar* et al., 1980] reported comparable results us-

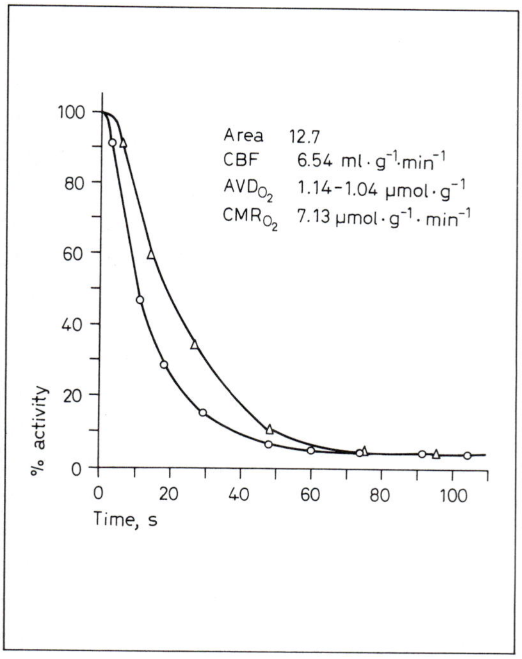

Fig. 2. Cerebral metabolism and neural function. Application of the *Kety and Schmidt* technique to high flow situation (hypercapnia). Note fast decrease in venous concentration of ^{133}Xenon (△) [Reproduced from *Berntman* et al.: Anesthesiology *50:* 299–305, 1979].

ing the ^{14}C-deoxyglucose technique of *Sokoloff* et al. [1977]. It should also be recalled that the ^{15}O-technique has yielded CMR_{O_2} figures in man, similar to those previously reported by workers using the *Kety and Schmidt* inert gas technique [*Raichle* et al., 1976].

Measurements of CMR_{O_2}

Limitations

There is no question that the main limitation of such measurements is the poor spatial resolution since the *Kety and Schmidt* technique either yields values for the whole brain (measurements in man with venous sampling from the jugular bulb) or the 'cerebral cortex' (measurements in animals with sampling from the superior sagittal sinus). A better spatial resolution is obtained with the ^{15}O method described by *Ter-Pogossian* et al. [1970] but satisfactory measurements of *regional* CMR_{O_2} can only be obtained when that principle is utilized in tomographic recording systems [see article by *Lenzi* et al., this symposium]. However, such measurements are only applicable to man, or to large experimental animals, and the resolution is inferior to that obtained in experimental animals with the ^{14}C-deoxyglucose technique.

Advantages

The advantages are of two types. First, measurements of CMR_{O_2} allow assessment of changes in metabolic rate with a better time resolution. Second, they yield a more accurate estimate of metabolic rate in situations accompanied by a mismatch between oxygen consumption and glucose utilization.

Time Resolution. At normal blood flow rates in the rat, the *Kety and Schmidt* technique requires a steady-state period of 5–10 min and, at greatly increased flow rates, this time is less than 5 min (fig. 2). These figures should be compared to the 30- to 45-min steady-state period required to assess local CMR_{gl}. Furthermore, when continuous venous outflow measurements are combined with measurements of arteriovenous differences in oxygen content semi-quantitative values for CMR_{O_2} can be obtained on a minute-to-minute basis [e.g. *Altenburg* et al., 1969; *Sari* et al., 1975; *Meldrum and Nilsson,* 1976; *Nilsson and Siesjö,* in press).

Table I. Comparison of local glucose consumption (CMR_{gl}) in frontal and parietal cortex and oxygen consumption (CMR_{O_2}) in animals ventilated on 70% N_2O or given 150 mg · kg^{-1} of phenobarbital

Anesthesia	CMR_{O_2} measured	CMR_{gl}	
		calculated	found
70% N_2	4.0	0.70	0.70
Phenobarbital 150 mg · kg^{-1}	2.7	0.47	0.32

Data from *Ingvar* et al. [1980].

Oxygen Consumption versus Glucose Utilization. Several conditions exist in which glucose utilization is either more or less than that which corresponds to oxygen consumption. One example is provided by starvation or other conditions in which ketone bodies account for part of the oxygen consumed by the brain. However, even more common are these conditions in which the rate of glycolysis is changed. For example, in the initial phases of hypoxia and epileptic seizures part of the glucose phosphorylated leads to accumulation of lactic acid. Clearly, in such conditions glucose utilization is in excess of the CMR_{O_2}. The reverse occurs in hypoglycemia, a condition in which lack of exogenous glucose leads to oxidation of endogenous carbohydrate and amino acid substrates. Accordingly, glucose utilization falls short of CMR_{O_2}. It has now been established that a similar situation, albeit of a less dramatic degree, occurs in hypercapnia and in barbiturate anesthesia. As an example, we can illustrate the correspondence between CMR_{O_2} and CMR_{gl} in rats maintained on 70% N_2O, and the lack of correspondence in those anesthetized with phenobarbital (table I). In all probability, the large reduction of CMR_{gl} in phenobarbital anesthesia (and in hypercapnia) is due to inhibition of glycolysis at the phosphofructokinase step. As a result, the reduced supply of carbon skeletons from glucose has to be compensated for by oxidation of endogenous carbohydrate substrates, and by mobilization of carbon skeletons from the amino acid pools [see *Folbergrová* et al., 1975; *Miller* et al., 1975; *Chapman* et al., 1978].

In summary, although measurements of local glucose consumption will be the dominant technique for measuring metabolic rate in the brain, measurements of CMR_{O_2} are indispensible for assessing rapid changes in metabolic rate, and for measuring metabolic rate in conditions causing a mismatch between oxygen consumption and glucose utilization.

Acknowledgements

Most of the work mentioned in this article from the author's own laboratory was supported by grants from the Swedish Medical Research Council and from NIH.

References

Alexander, S.C.; Wollman, H.; Cohen, P.J.; Chase, P.E.; Melman, E.; Behar, M.: ^{85}Kr and nitrous oxide uptake of the human brain during anesthesia. Anesthesiology *25:* 37–42 (1964).

Altenburg, B.M.; Michenfelder, J.D.; Theye, R.A.: Acute tolerance to thiopental in canine cerebral oxygen consumption studies. Anesthesiology *31:* 443–448 (1969).

Chapman, A.G.; Nordström, C.-H.; Siesjö, B.K.: Influence of phenobarbital anaesthesia on carbohydrate and amino acid metabolism in rat brain. Anesthesiology *48:* 175–182 (1978).

Folbergrová, J.; Norberg, K.; Quistorff, B.; Siesjö, B.K.: Carbohydrate and amino acid metabolism in rat cerebral cortex in moderate and extreme hypercapnia. J. Neurochem. *25:* 457–462 (1975).

Homburger, E.; Himwich, W.A.; Etsten, B.; York, G.; Maresca, R.; Himwich, H.E.: Effect of pentothal anesthesia on canine cerebral cortex. Am. J. Physiol. *147:* 343–345 (1946).

Ingvar, M.; Abdul-Rahman, A.; Siesjö, B.K.: Local cerebral glucose consumption in the artificially ventilated rat: influence of nitrous oxide analgesia and of phenobarbital anesthesia. Acta physiol. scand. *109:* 177–185 (1980).

Kety, S.S.; Schmidt, C.F.: The nitrous oxide method for the quantitative determination of cerebral blood flow in man: theory, procedure and normal values. J. clin. Invest. *27:* 476–483 (1948).

Lassen, N.A.; Klee, A.: Cerebral blood flow determined by saturation and desaturation with Krypton^{85}: an evaluation of the validity of the inert gas method of Kety and Schmidt. Circulation Res. *16:* 26–32 (1965).

Lassen, N.A.; Munck, O.: The cerebral blood flow in man determined by the use of radioactive krypton. Acta physiol. scand. *33:* 30–49 (1955).

McHenry, L.C., Jr.: Determination of cerebral blood flow by a krypton-85 desaturation method. Nature, Lond. *200:* 1297–1299 (1963).

Meldrum, B.; Nilsson, B.: Cerebral blood flow and metabolic rate early and late in prolonged epileptic seizures induced in rats by bicuculline. Brain *99:* 523–542 (1976).

Michenfelder, J.D.; Messick, J.M., Jr.; Theye, R.A.: Simultaneous cerebral blood flow measured by direct and indirect methods. J. surg. Res. *8:* 475–481 (1968).

Miller, A.L.; Hawkins, R.A.; Veech, R.L.: Decreased rate of glucose utilization by rat brain in vivo after exposures to atmospheres containing high concentrations of CO_2. J. Nerochem. *25:* 553–558 (1975).

Nilsson, B.; Siesjö, B.K.: A method for determining blood flow and oxygen consumption in the rat brain. Acta physiol. scand. *96:* 72–82 (1976).

Nilsson, B.; Siesjö, B.K.: A venous outflow method for measurement of rapid changes of the cerebral blood flow and oxygen consumption in the rat. Stroke (in press).

Norberg, K.; Siesjö, B.K.: Oxidative metabolism of the cerebral cortex of the rat in severe insulin-induced hypoglycemia. J. Neurochem. *26:* 345–352 (1976).

Raichle, M.E.; Grubb, R.L., Jr.; Eichling, J.O.; Ter-Pogossian, M.M.: Measurement of brain oxygen utilization with radioactive oxygen-15: experimental verifications. J. appl. Physiol. *40:* 638–640 (1976).

Sari, A.; Fukuda, Y.; Sakabe, T.; Maekawa, T.; Ishikawa, T.: Effects of psychotropic drugs on canine cerebral metabolism and circulation related to EEG – diazepam, clomipramine, and chlorpromazine. J. Neurol. Neurosurg. Psychiat. *38:* 838–844 (1975).

Siesjö, B.K.: Brain energy metabolism (Wiley, Chichester 1978).

Siesjö, B.K.; Berntman, L.; Nilsson, B.: Blood flow and oxygen consumption using the Kety-Schmidt technique; in Passenneau, Hawkins, Lust, Welsh, Cerebral metabolism and neural function, pp. 223–232 (Williams & Wilkins, Baltimore 1980).

Sokoloff, L.; Reivich, M.; Kennedy, C.; Des Rosiers, M.H.; Patlak, C.; Pettigrew, K.; Sakurada, O.; Shinohara, M.: The ^{14}C-deoxyglycose method for the measurement of local cerebral glucose utilization. J. Neurochem. *28:* 897–916 (1977).

Ter-Pogossian, M.M.; Eichling, J.O.; Davis, D.W.; Welch, M.J.: The measure in vivo of regional cerebral oxygen utilization by means of oxyhemoglobin labeled with radioactive oxygen-15. J. clin. Invest. *49:* 381–391 (1963).

Bo K. Siesjö, Laboratory of Experimental Brain Research, University Hospital, S–221 85 Lund (Sweden)

Eur. Neurol. *20:* 200–206 (1981)

Determination of Tissular pO_2 in Brain Microvascular Research

Usefulness and Limitations

N. Wiernsperger, P. Gygax

Preclinical Research, Sandoz Ltd., Basel, Switzerland

Key Words. Tissue pO_2 · Microcirculation · Brain ischemia · Brain metabolism · Drugs

Abstract. Principles of O_2 delivery to the brain as well as basic technological description of tissue pO_2 measurement are described. Examples of application of the pO_2 technique to vascular or metabolic disorders of the brain show that tissue pO_2 is a remarkable indicator for microcirculatory disturbances. It is shown that pO_2 is the most local parameter available in microcirculatory research. Therefore, it provides useful information about the quality of capillary perfusion. However, as pO_2 is a resultant of many factors involved in the regulation of microcirculation, limitations exist in the interpretation of the data, which are discussed.

Introduction

Oxygen is delivered to tissues by diffusion from the blood. This occurs by passive diffusion along two gradients, along and across to the vessel axis [6]. However, these gradients are modulated by the blood flow direction, depending on whether the blood flows parallel or counter to adjacent capillaries. Therefore, a three-dimensional distribution of tissue partial oxygen pressure (pO_2) takes place, resulting in a so-called oxygen pressure field. Whereas the oxygen supply to the tissue is relatively simple in capillary beds with a parallel arrangement of capillaries (skeletal muscle), it is rather complicated in network structures like the capillaries of the brain [2]. The brain is supplied with blood by an extremely dense capillary network, the total length of capillaries within 1 mm^3 cortex being about 40 cm [10]. Furthermore, a high number of connections between the capillaries allows very localized adjustments of the microcirculation within the network. It therefore appears that, due to the architecture of the microvessels, a great variation in O_2 delivery to the tissue will be found, depending on the site of the measurement. Other factors also influence the oxygen supply to the tissue: the arterial oxygen blood content, the cerebral blood flow, tissue metabolism, rheological properties of blood, the diffusion coefficient for oxygen in a given tissue. From this brief description, it is apparent that the regulation of O_2 supply occurs in restricted areas. Thus, the measurement of tissue oxygenation represents the most local determination of microcirculatory events that can be achieved with presently available techniques. Moreover, tissue oxygenation can be regarded as the result of all factors influencing the microcirculation and thus is a direct indicator of the level of perfusion of the capillary bed.

The technique used for pO_2 determination is based on the principles of polarography. By applying a negative potential to the electrode, O_2 present in the medium is reduced according to the equation of *Kolthoff and Lingane* [5]. The reduction needs four electrons per molecule, giving rise to a current which can be measured and is directly proportional to the O_2 pressure at the tip of the electrode. As the tissue pO_2 varies within distances of a few micrometers, the electrode tip must be as small as possible in order to avoid an integration over a wide tissue area. This also avoids mechanical compression of the capillary bed. An extensive description of all technical aspects of the pO_2 method can be found in the book by *Fatt* [1]. The following methodological heading therefore only concerns the technique used in the experiments to be described.

Methods

Two different types of pO_2 microelectrodes have been used. For recordings within the cortical tissue, gold microelectrodes were constructed. They consisted of a gold wire, which was threaded in a glass capillary, leaving a tip of 1 mm length free for insertion into the tissue. After abrading the gold wire on diamond paste, the tip (2–3 μm diameter) was coated with an oxygen-permeable membrane. Surface electrodes were constructed by melting an etched, chemically pure platinum wire (tip diameter: 1–2 μm) with glass, polishing the glass with abrasive paper and applying a polystyrol membrane as above.

pO_2 measurements were achieved by applying a potential of −700 mV for platinum and −1,000 mV for gold electrodes against a silver-silver chloride reference electrode. For details of the electronic circuitry see *Wiernsperger* et al. [11]. The electrodes were calibrated for minimal and maximal pO_2 by dipping in a glucose-glucose oxidase solution and in air-equilibrated physiological saline at 37 °C, respectively. This procedure was repeated at the end of the experiment and, in the case of surface elements, at intervals during the experiment.

Biological Applications of the pO_2 Technique

Tissular pO_2 Studies in Vascular Disorders of the Brain

Hypovolemic Oligemia

The studies were performed on N_2O/O_2 anesthetized cats which were immobilized and artificially ventilated. Blood pressure was lowered below the limit of autoregulation by bleeding the animals to a mean arterial blood pressure (MABP) of 45 mm Hg. The pO_2 measurements were made in the suprasylvian gyrus of the left hemisphere by using gold and platinum microelectrodes. Regional cerebral blood flow (rCBF) was determined by the local hydrogen clearance technique in the same area of the cortex. The EEG was recorded in the frontoparietal region and analyzed on-line by Fourier transformation.

The oligemic state was characterized by a drastic decrease in tissue pO_2 which is seen as a leftward shift in the histogram. Such a profile is typical for tissue hypoxia (fig. 1a). At the same time, rCBF and the EEG were depressed [13].

The attempt to correct this situation by increasing the CBF with papaverine (1 mg/kg i.v.) led to a dissociation of the pO_2 histo-

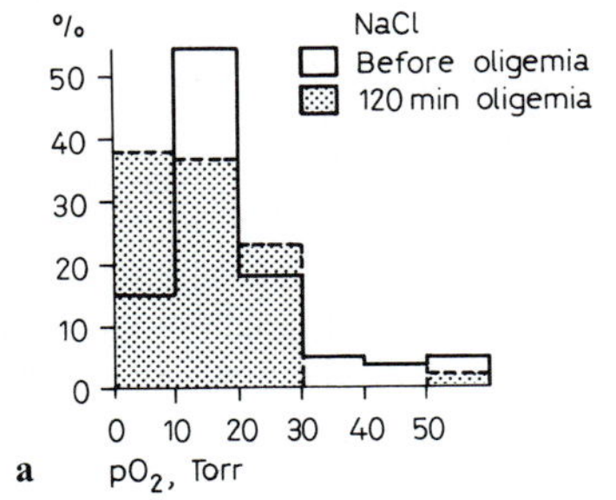

Fig. 1. a Tissue pO_2 distribution in cat cerebral cortex under normotensive and oligemic conditions.

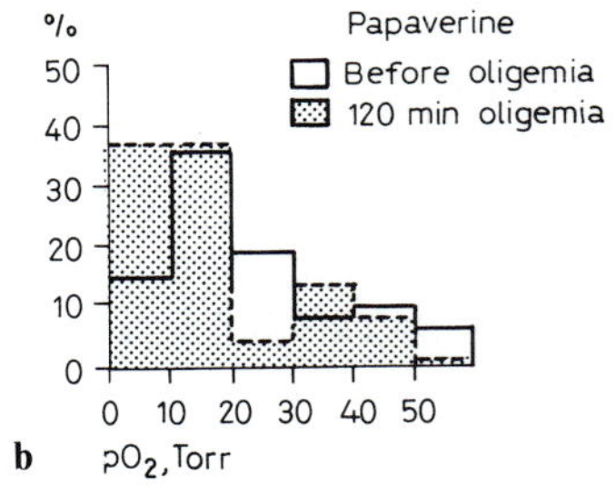

b Effect of papaverine (1 mg/kg i.v.) on cortical pO_2 distribution under oligemic conditions.

gram into two groups (fig. 1b). Whereas the majority of the pO_2 values remained low, a group of high values could still be registered. At this time, the rCBF, in spite of being measured locally, indicated an increase in perfusion. However, no improvement in the EEG could be seen following papaverine administration [12]. The bimodal profile of the histogram characterizes an uneven distribution of microflow, some areas being overperfused at the expense of other, underperfused regions. Thus, through its high resolution, the pO_2 technique allowed the detection of shunting effects in the microcirculation of microareas of tissue, which could not be detected even with the most local CBF method.

However, the use of pO_2 determinations has limitations. This can be illustrated in the following example. The cerebral perfusion under oligemic conditions was increased using apomorphine (2 mg/kg i.v.). This resulted in an apparent increase in EEG power, the detailed analysis of which revealed that the preservation of high power values was due to an enhancement of oligemia-induced seizures [13]. On the other hand, a complete normalization of the pO_2 distribution could be registered (fig. 2). In this case, and in contrast to other drugs [12], the normalized tissue oxygenation was not accompanied by an improvement in brain electrical function. Consideration of only pO_2 histograms can thus be misleading.

Vasospasm

Vasospasm is a common complication in stroke and is often difficult to visualize with angiographic techniques. Vasospasm can be induced experimentally by superfusing the brain with blood or plasma. The cortex of cats was superfused with autologous platelet-poor plasma for 30 min [15]. There was no apparent bleaching of the cortex. Nevertheless, a marked decrease in tissue pO_2 was observed, illustrated by a shift to the left in the histogram (fig. 3).

The morphometric analysis of the capillaries revealed a reduction in the lumen of precapillary fragments as well as of real capillaries, thus limiting the amount of blood and oxygen available for the tissue [15]. The fact that a complete reversal of tissue hypoxia

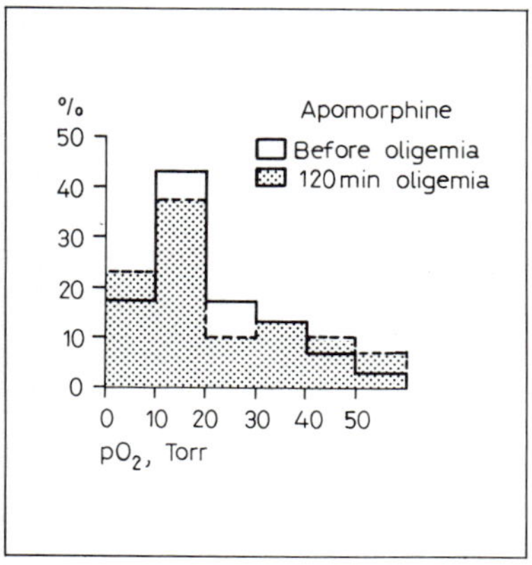

Fig. 2. Effect of apomorphine (2 mg/kg i.v.) on cortical pO_2 distribution under oligemic conditions.

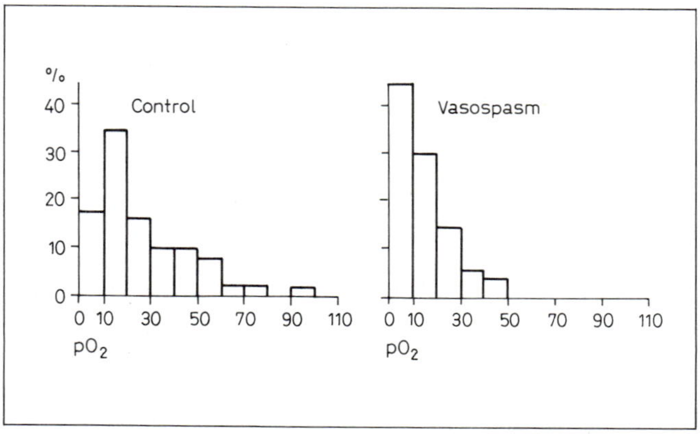

Fig. 3. Effect of vasospasm induced by platelet-poor plasma on the cortical pO_2 distribution in cats.

could be obtained after treatment with the Ca^{++} antagonist nifedipine (0.02 mg/kg) indicated that the constriction of the microvessels was not simply due to a passive adaptation to the low flow state, but that active contraction mechanisms were involved in the spastic process (fig. 4).

In an attempt to overcome the vascular constriction, the MABP was raised by slow infusion of the adrenergic drug Effortil®. Whereas control animals invariably showed an increase in tissue pO_2, the spastic animals showed either stable, elevated or decreased pO_2 values. Furthermore, a tendency for edema to develop was seen in animals with vasospasm. These findings illustrate a patchy distribution of the microflow, depending on the resistance of the different microvascular beds [15]. In this model, the pO_2 measurements provided the first demonstration of changes in the *micro*circulation of the cortex under conditions of acute vasospasm. Moreover, the method allowed us to observe redistribution phenomena of microflow within small areas of tissue following a blood pressure increasing therapy.

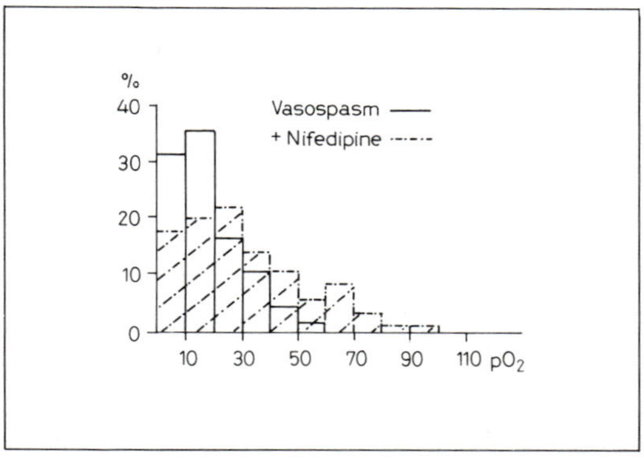

Fig. 4. Reversal of vasospasm-induced tissue hypoxia by treatment with the Ca^{++} antagonist nifedipine (0.02 mg/kg i.v.) in rabbits.

Focal Cerebral Ischemia

In N_2O/O_2 anesthetized cats, a small branch of the middle cerebral artery was clamped onto the ectosylvian gyrus with a neurosurgical microclip. The pO_2 measurements were done by placing a surface pO_2 electrode in the supplying area of an arteriole derived from the MCA branch. Gold microelectrodes were placed in the immediate vicinity of the surface electrode. After 45 min

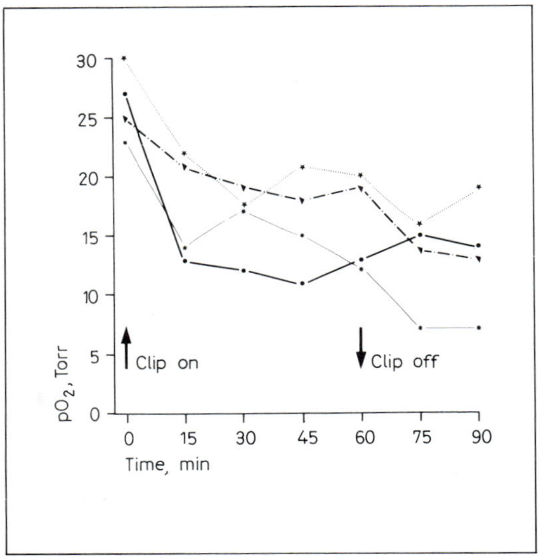

Fig. 5. Effect of focal ischemia induced by arterial clamping on tissular pO_2 of cat cortex (four representative original tracings are shown). Note the further decrease in tissue pO_2 after removal of the clip.

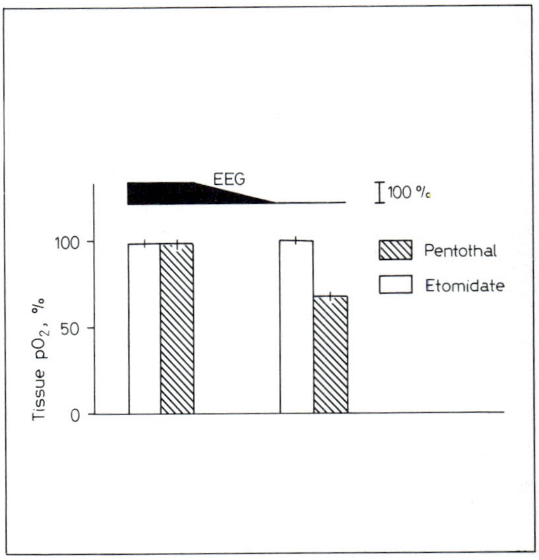

Fig. 6. Effect of anesthetics (pentothal and Etomidate) on cortical tissue pO_2. In contrast to pentothal, tissular pO_2 remains normal when the EEG is flat.

occlusion, the clip was removed to allow the reperfusion of the ischemic zone. The pO_2 tracings showed that occlusion led to an immediate decrease in tissue pO_2 (fig. 5). The size of the ischemic area was estimated to be in the order of 3–4 mm^2, as the electrodes placed around the surface element showed no reaction to the occlusion.

After removing the clip, a further decrease in tissue pO_2 was observed in most cases, which could not be overcome by increasing the MABP. In this model, pO_2 measurements were of special usefulness, as the ischemic area was very restricted and therefore required measurements as localized as possible. They showed that the no-reflow phenomena, the existence of which is debated, can be encountered in most cases of postischemic reperfusion of brain tissue in our experimental situation.

Tissue pO_2 and Reduced Brain Metabolism

Glucose consumption was reduced in the brain by pharmacological manipulation of the tissue metabolism. Pentothal or Etomidate® were infused in cats in cumulative doses until the EEG became completely flat. The reaction of the tissue oxygenation to this extreme reduction of metabolic demand was measured by inserting several gold electrodes into the parietal cortex. While no change was seen with Etomidate, a decrease in tissue pO_2 was observed with pentothal (fig. 6). The latter decrease could be compensated by increasing the systemic blood pressure, which indicates that barbiturates interfere with CBF. The maintenance of a normal tissue oxygen level with Etomidate should make this drug more suitable for neurosurgical interventions than barbiturates.

Conclusions

Theoretical considerations of the microcirculation in the brain make the tissular pO_2 one of the most interesting parameters which can be measured, because it represents the resultant of a multifactorial mechanism of microflow control. Due to the anatomical arrangement of the microvessels in the brain, there is an extensive heterogeneity in tissue oxygenation which ranges from almost zero to the arterial oxygen value. Most adaptive mechanisms of microflow occur within discrete tissue areas and therefore cannot be detected by classical methods of blood flow measurement. For these reasons, the evaluation of tissue oxygenation not only requires a very local technique with high resolution (10–15 μm), but also has to be performed in most cases by the determination of the entire oxygen pressure field. It is evident that a single pO_2 measurement at one site yields only minor information. Therefore, the state of an organ has to be analyzed by oxygen distribution profiles, i.e. histograms [4].

The microelectrode technique fulfils these requirements. The method is very local and extremely sensitive (0.5 mm Hg). Applications in brain research show that tissue pO_2 is a remarkable indicator of even slight and limited changes in the microcirculation. An illustrative example has been given in the studies concerning hypovolemic oligemia, where extremely local inhomogeneities of microflow could be seen in spite of an apparent increase in cerebral blood flow. The pO_2 measurements are of special use in cases of blood flow redistribution within the capillary network (hypovolemic oligemia, vasospasm, ...). They also allow one to follow the development of oxygen insufficiency with time. Therefore, they should find a useful application in neurosurgery [9]. Finally, pO_2 measurements discriminate between the pharmacological actions of drugs [3, 8]. These characteristics make the pO_2 technique one of the most reliable methods available for microcirculatory research.

However, there are some limitations to the application and interpretation of the method. Not only is the construction of the microelectrodes time-consuming, but their use is theoretically limited to outer structures of the brain like the cortex, as far as distribution studies are concerned. On the other hand, tissular pO_2 is strongly influenced by metabolic factors. However, it is not a direct indicator of oxygen consumption, as other factors interfere with the tissue O_2 level (blood flow, nervous and chemical factors, hemorheological factors). The single consideration of tissue pO_2 could lead to false interpretations, as has been demonstrated for the effect of apomorphine in case of hypovolemic oligemia [13]. An apparently correct tissue oxygenation in no way means that the function of the organ is guaranteed. It just represents a necessary condition for oxygen-requiring biochemical reactions to proceed. Therefore, whenever possible, the pO_2 technique should be used in combination with other methods such as cerebral blood flow measurements, EEG or ion selective electrodes.

References

1 Fatt, I.: Polarographic oxygen sensors (CRC Press, 1976).

2 Grunewald, W.A.; Sowa, W.: Capillary structures and O_2 supply to tissue. Rev. Physiol. Biochem. Pharmacol. *77:* 150–209 (1977).

3 Gygax, P.; Wiernsperger, N.: The significance of pO_2 histograms in CNS pharmacology. Arzneimittel-Forsch. (in press).

4 Kessler, M.; Höper, J.; Krumme, B.A.: Monitoring of tissue perfusion and cellular function. Anesthesiology *45:* 184–197 (1976).
5 Kolthoff, J.M.; Lingane, J.J.: Polarography (Interscience, New York 1952).
6 Krogh, A.: The number and distribution of capillaries in muscles with calculations of the oxygen pressure head necessary for supplying the tissue. J. Physiol., Lond. *52:* 409–415 (1918–1919).
7 Metzger, H.: Verteilung des O_2-Partialdrucks im Mikrobereich des Gehirngewebes. Polarographische Messung und mathematische Analyse; Habschr. Mainz (1971).
8 Plotkine, M.; Paultre, C.Z.; Boulu, R.; Rossignol, P.: Intérêt pharmacologique d'une technique d'enregistrement de la pO_2 tissulaire du cortex cérébral chez le lapin. Réponse à la papavérine et au naftidrofuryl. Thérapie *30:* 713–723 (1975).
9 Silver, I.A.: The significance of clinical assessment of brain oxygenation in different pathological conditions: an overview. Fed. Proc. *38:* 2495–2500 (1979).
10 Wiederhold, K.H.; Bielser, W.; Schulz, U.; Veteau, M.J.; Hunziker, O.: Three-dimensional reconstruction of brain capillaries from frozen serial sections. Microvasc. Res. *11:* 175–180 (1976).
11 Wiernsperger, N.; Kunke, S.; Gygax, P.: Technical note about simultaneous recording of oxygen partial pressure and neuronal activity in cat cortex. Experientia *32:* 671–673 (1976).
12 Wiernsperger, N.; Gygax, P.; Danzeisen, M.: Cortical pO_2 distribution during oligemic hypotension and its pharmacological modifications. Arzneimittel-Forsch. *28:* 768–770 (1978).
13 Wiernsperger, N.; Gygax, P.; Schweizer, A.; Danzeisen, M.: Dopaminergic agonists and their influence on the oxygenation and functional activity of underperfused brain tissue. Eur. J. Pharmacol. *60:* 115–119 (1979).
14 Wiernsperger, N.; Gygax, P.; Meier-Ruge, W.; Danzeisen, M.: Improvement of brain tissue oxygenation during cerebrovascular insufficiency by interfering with the catecholaminergic system. Biblthca anat., vol. 18, pp. 161–163 (Karger, Basel 1979).
15 Wiernsperger, N.; Schulz, U.; Gygax, P.: Physiological and morphometrical analysis of the microcirculation in the cerebral cortex under acute vasospasm (in press).

N. Wiernsperger, Preclinical Research,
Sandoz Ltd., CH–4000 Basel (Switzerland)

Eur. Neurol. *20:* 207–214 (1981)

An Introduction to the Measurement of the Cerebral Oxygen Uptake Rate by Inhalation of $^{15}O_2$: Analysis of the Contribution of $^{15}O_2$ and $H_2{}^{15}O$ in Brain Radioactivity

J.C. Depresseux[a], *M.E. Raichle*[b], *K.B. Larson*[c], *J. Markham*[c], *M.M. Ter-Pogossian*[b]

[a]National Foundation for Scientific Research, Cyclotron Research Center, University of Liège, Liège, Belgium; [b]Division of Radiation Sciences, Edward Mallinckrodt Institute of Radiology, Department of Neurology and of Neurological Surgery, and [c]Biomedical Computing Laboratory, Washington University School of Medicine, St. Louis, Mo., USA

Key Words. Brain · $^{15}O_2$ · Model · Water metabolism

Abstract. This paper introduces a model for the computation of the regional cerebral metabolic rate of oxygen from the data of cerebral regional radioactivity collected after inhalation of $^{15}O_2$. A method was devised for the differential determination of the respective contribution of radiooxygen and of radiowater in the inflow and the outflow of radioactivity in the brain after or during such on inhalation. The results demonstrate the feasability of such a model and outline some of the methodological prerequisites to be taken into account in the numerical analysis of the data.

Introduction

The design of a method for the determination of the regional cerebral metabolic rate of oxygen (CMR_{O_2}) in man encounters several difficulties, mainly linked to the impossibility of conceiving a method using an analogue of oxygen, to the rapid physical decay of $^{15}O_2$ and to the high rate at which oxydoreduction processes occur in the tissues, especially in the brain.

The classical technique of *Kety and Schmidt* [1] yields only a measurement of global CMR_{O_2} and affords no idea on the spatial distribution of this parameter in physiological and physiopathological conditions.

The method using a sequential intracarotid injection of $^{15}O_2$ and of $H_2{}^{15}O$, with regional external counting of the cerebral activity [2] is presently the only technique for measuring regional values of CMR_{O_2} in man. Its application to human beings is still limited by the necessity of a carotid access.

The present research was done in view of defining the prerequisites of a model for the numerical analysis of regional cerebral activities detected after inhalation of $^{15}O_2$. The high rate of oxygen diffusion and reduction in the brain makes one of the first problems to be encountered the contribution of radiowater in the inflow and in the outflow of radioactivity in each detection area of the brain.

Methods

Experimental Setup

The time course of the $^{15}O_2$ and $H_2{}^{15}O$ activity in the internal carotid artery and in the internal jugular vein blood after a bolus inhalation of $^{15}O_2$ was determined in 3 adult baboons and in 2 rhesus monkeys, prepared by ligation of the branches of the external carotid arteries. The monkeys were paralyzed with gallamine and passively ventilated with an anesthetizing mixture $N_2O(70\%)$–$O_2(30\%)$. End-tidal pCO_2, arterial blood pressure and rectal temperature were continuously monitored. Temperature was maintained between 37 and 39 °C with a heating pad.

Blood was sampled from one internal carotid artery and from the ipsilateral jugular vein through small catheters positioned under fluoroscopic control from the femoral artery.

After a bolus inhalation of $^{15}O_2$, carotid and jugular blood are sampled during 120 s. The radioactivity is separately measured on the total blood and on the corresponding plasma phase of each sample. Any loss of $^{15}O_2$ is avoided by handling blood under a protective oil film. Volumes of samples are measured by weighing. Countings are corrected for physical decay. A continuous withdrawal of blood through the catheters was maintained during the whole sampling procedure and the time shift between the activity in the vessels and in the samples was verified to be negligible.

Arterial pO_2, hemoglobin concentration, hematocrit, pH and pCO_2 were measured before and after each inhalation of labeled oxygen.

The cerebral blood flow (CBF) was measured by rapid injection of $H_2{}^{15}O$-labeled blood into the internal carotid artery and by detection of the radioactivity of the head with a 3 × 2 in NaI(Tl) scintillation detector, following the method of *Ter-Pogossian* et al. [2]. CMR_{O_2} was computed by multiplying CBF by the cerebral arteriovenous difference in oxygen blood content.

Determination of $^{15}O_2$ and of $H_2{}^{15}O$ Activities in the Blood

The differential determination of $^{15}O_2$ and $H_2{}^{15}O$ radioactivities in the blood are based on dual counting on the whole blood and on the plasma phase and on a data processing based on the knowledge of the distribution of oxygen and water in erythrocytes and plasma at equilibrium. Oxygen is distributed in three compartments, oxyhemoglobin, dissolved oxygen in erythrocytes and dissolved oxygen in plasma, and water is distributed in two compartments, erythrocytes and plasma.

Equations 1, 2 and 3 can be written, with the following symbols: C values are quantities per unit volume of whole blood, erythrocytes or plasma, as indicated by the subscripts b, e and p; diss O_2, HbO_2 and H_2O indicate dissolved oxygen, hemoglobin-linked oxygen and water, respectively; α_eO_2 is the Bunsen coefficient of solubility of oxygen in erythrocytes at 37 °C; α_pO_2 is the corresponding coefficient for plasma; pO_2 is the partial pressure of oxygen in blood in Torr; H is the hematocrit value; C_{O_2} is the oxygen content of the blood, as oxyhemoglobin, expressed as [ml O_2(NTP)] × [ml whole blood]$^{-1}$; λ was experimentally measured by the measurement of the distribution of $H_2{}^{15}O$ between red cells and plasma.

$$k \triangleq \frac{C_{e\,diss\,O_2}}{C_{eHbO_2}} = \frac{\alpha_eO_2 \times pO_2 \times H}{C_{O_2}}, \tag{1}$$

$$\gamma \triangleq \frac{C_{p\,diss\,O_2}}{C_{e\,diss\,O_2}} = \frac{\alpha_pO_2}{\alpha_eO_2} = 0.81, \tag{2}$$

$$\lambda \triangleq \frac{C_{eH_2O}}{C_{pH_2O}} = 0.81. \tag{3}$$

The value of α_eO_2 is 3.39 × 10^{-5} [ml O_2(NPT)] × [ml erythrocyte]$^{-1}$ × [Torr.]$^{-1}$; the value of α_pO_2 is 2.75 × 10^{-5} [ml O_2(NPT)] × [ml plasma]$^{-1}$ × [Torr]$^{-1}$ [3]; pO_2 and pH are measured on blood sample; C_{O_2} is determined from pO_2, pH and the concentration in hemoglobin of the blood.

The equilibrium distribution of $^{15}O_2$ and $H_2{}^{15}O$ may be assumed to be the same as that of unlabeled oxygen and water in the blood, and the above-mentioned equations be applied, with C values indicating activites per unit volume.

The activities of O_2 and H_2O in each of the five compartments can be calculated from the measurement of C_b, the activity of whole blood in cps × [ml whole blood]$^{-1}$ and C_p, the activity of the corresponding plasma phase, in cps × [ml plasma]$^{-1}$.

$$C_{eHbO_2} = \frac{C_b - (1 - H + \lambda H)\, C_p}{H\,(1 + k - \lambda kv)}, \qquad (4)$$

$$C_{e\,diss\,O_2} = kC_{eHbO_2}, \qquad (5)$$

$$C_{p\,diss\,O_2} = kvC_{eHbO_2}, \qquad (6)$$

$$C_{pH_2O} = C_p - C_{p\,diss\,O_2}, \qquad (7)$$

$$C_{eH_2O} = \lambda C_{pH_2O}. \qquad (8)$$

The values of interest, radio oxygen and radio water concentrations in the blood, are finally computed as follows, expressed as cps × [ml whole blood]$^{-1}$.

$$C_{bO_2} = HC_{eHbO_2} + HC_{e\,diss\,O_2} + (1-H)\, C_{p\,diss\,O_2} \qquad (9)$$

$$C_{bH_2O} = HC_{eH_2O} + (1-H)\, C_{pH_2O} \qquad (10)$$

The errors resulting from the aleatory character of radioactive decay are also estimated.

The application of these equations to blood samples labeled in vitro only with $^{15}O_2$ or $H_2{}^{15}O$ yielded values for C_{bH_2O} and C_{bO_2} which were, respectively, not significantly different from zero, thus validating the method.

Results and Discussion

Rationale of the Study

The measurement of regional uptake rate of oxygen in the brain has been carried out from the externally detected activity on the head after rapid and sequential injection of $^{15}O_2$ and of $H_2{}^{15}O$ in the internal carotid artery [2]. This method has been thoroughly validated [4–6] and applied to physiological and physiopathological studies [7, 8]. The application of this reference method is still limited by the ethical impediment of performing and, especially, repeating a carotid artery puncture in most patients.

Methods proceeding by inhalation instead of arterial injection of oxygen were consequently investigated, either with bolus inhalation of $^{15}O_2$ and detection by probes [9] or with sequential continuous breathing of $^{15}O_2$ and C $^{15}O_2$ and detection by positron emission tomography (PET) [10, 11].

As the intracarotid method [2] measures the extraction fraction of $^{15}O_2$ by the brain from the detection of the first capillary transit of the tracer in the tissue, the data which are taken into account are not altered by any interference of $H_2{}^{15}O$ activity, however rapid the reduction of $^{15}O_2$ may be.

On the contrary, if the administration of $^{15}O_2$ is spread more over time and if the detection data are collected during a longer period of time, the contribution of metabolically produced $H_2{}^{15}O$ is to be taken into account in the analysis of the results.

Inflow and Outflow of Labeled Oxygen and Water in the Brain

Figure 1 illustrates that $H_2{}^{15}O$ activity rises in the arterial and jugular blood very early after the oxygen inhalation, in connection with the high rate at which oxygen is metabolically reduced in the tissues and with the relatively small tissular oxygen pool. Thus the arterial activity, the inflow of which is to be considered in the analysis of externally detected cerebral activity, is built up with a mixture of radiooxygen and of radiowater from the earliest tens of seconds after the inhalation of $^{15}O_2$. The integral – from 0 up to 120 s – arterial radiowater activity ranged from 14.0 to 29.6% of the total blood activity in our observations. The jugular vein activity also shows the outflow of radiowater from the encephalus, the difference of $H_2{}^{15}O$ activities between the arterial and the venous sides depending on the cerebral production and back diffusion of labeled metabolic water.

Simulation of a Modeled Determination of CMR_{O_2}

The determination of the time course of the arterial and venous $^{15}O_2$ and $H_2{}^{15}O$ activities after a bolus inhalation of $^{15}O_2$ provides orientation data in order to specify the prerequisites of a model for the quantitative analysis of the externally detected brain activity after such an inhalation.

The calculation of CMR_{O_2} is conceivably accessible from the data of a sufficiently rapid PET [12] after a bolus inhalation of $^{15}O_2$, with the aid of a model describing oxygen tissular kinetics and of a numerical analysis technique derived from the published method for the measurement of regional substrate utilization rates by emission tomography [13]. This general model deals with tracers chemically identical to the studied substrates, with metabolic processes in which the tracee is in a steady state during the time of data collection and, finally, with systems in which no back diffusion of labeled metabolites occurs during the period under concern. The equation yielding, quite generally Φ, the estimated metabolic rate of the substrate, expressed as [mass substrate] $\times$ [unit time]$^{-1}$ $\times$ [unit mass tissue]$^{-1}$, is as follows

$$\Phi = \frac{q(t) - q_b(t)}{\int_0^t a_b(u)du + \frac{a_i(t)}{k(\alpha-1)}} \qquad (11)$$

where q(t) is the radioactivity in 1 PET element at time t, calibrated in [activity] $\times$ [unit mass tissue]$^{-1}$; $q_b(t)$ is the intravascular contribution in this activity; $a_b(u)$ is the specific activity of the tracer in the capillary blood of the studied region, expressed as [activity] $\times$ [unit mass tracee]$^{-1}$; $a_i(t)$ is the corresponding specific activity of the unmetabolized tracer in the extravascular space; α is the ratio between forward and reverse fluxes of the tracee across the capillary wall, and k is the ratio between the above-mentioned forward flux and the quantity of free tracee in the extravascular space, it is expressed as [unit time]$^{-1}$.

The application and the possible adaptation of this model to the measurement of CMR_{O_2} can be approached, using data derived from the observation in the monkey: the knowledge of the time course of the arterial and venous activities of $^{15}O_2$ and of $H_2{}^{15}O$, together with the cerebral blood flow, allow to compute simulated PET data to be fed in equation 11 or in a modified version of it and so to test the possibility of accurately computing CMR_{O_2} by this method.

The following points can be successively considered.

(1) As far as oxygen kinetics in the brain is concerned, the second term in the denominator of equation 11 has a negligible value, because α and k are high and because $a_i(t)$ is low and vanishes with time. In the present observation, α computed value is 14.75 and k estimation ranges between 8.1 and 41.1 s^{-1} when the apparent extravascular diffusion space allotted to oxygen varies from 76 to 15% of the tissular mass.

(2) The back diffusion and the circulatory washout of radiowater from the brain, the early occurrence of which is demonstrated in the present study, leads to an underestimation of PET data, q(t), in the numerator of equation 11. The value of the numerator is to be increased with an additional variable, $q_w(t)$ which contributes the net loss of radioactivity from the detected region at time t, i.e. the brain produced radiowater having left the region at time t (equation 12). Values for $q_w(t)$ can be computed from the cerebral blood flow and from the activity of $H_2{}^{15}O$ in the arterial and venous blood (fig. 2).

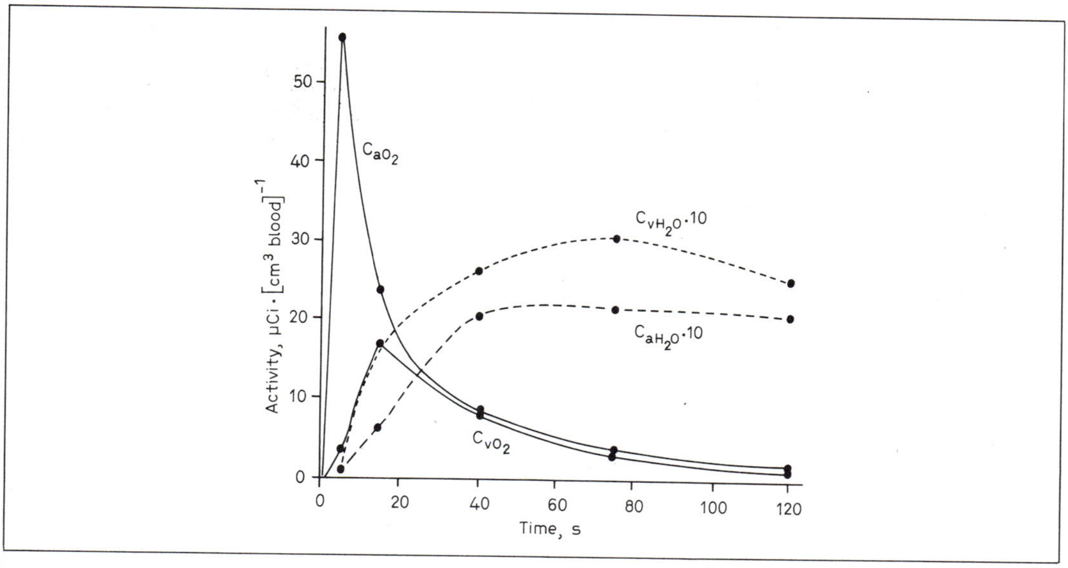

1

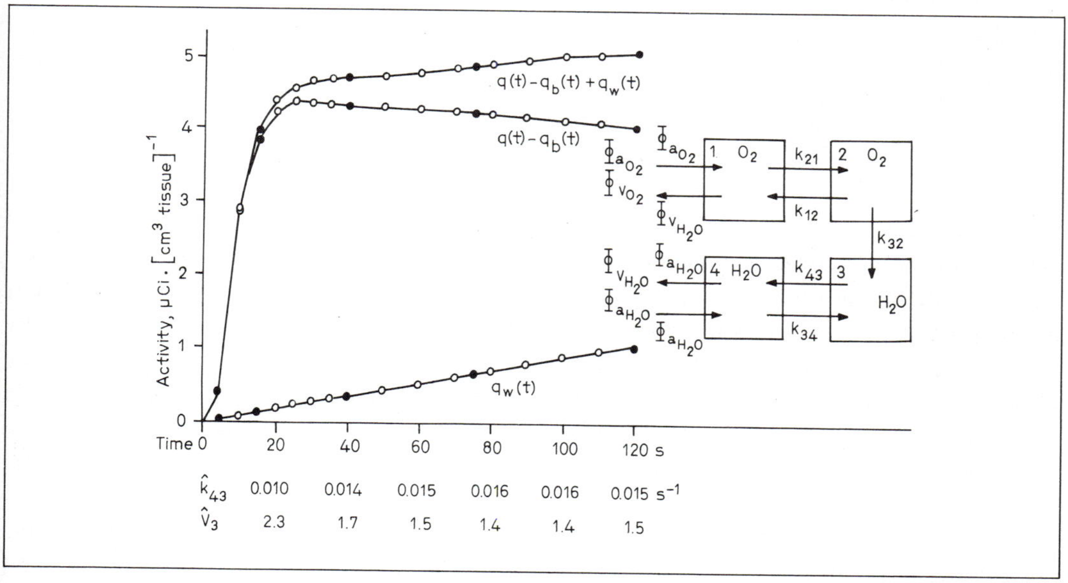

2

Fig. 1. An example of the time course of $^{15}O_2$ and $H_2{}^{15}O$ activities in carotid artery and in jugular vein of a baboon, after bolus inhalation of $^{15}O_2$. $H_2{}^{15}O$ metabolism appears very rapidly in the arterial and the cerebral venous blood.

Fig. 2. Simulated PET data (differential form) after inhalation of a bolus of $^{15}O_2$. q(t) is the total activity per unit volume of tissue at time t; $q_b(t)$ is the corresponding intravascular activity of $^{15}O_2$; $q_w(t)$ is the net loss of activity of brain-produced radiowater at time t. Inset: Tentative model for the description of the washout of radiowater from the brain with compartment 1, the intravascular oxygen; compartment 2, the extravascular oxygen; compartment 3, the extravascular metabolically produced water; compartment 4, the intravascular water. Estimations of k_{43} and of V_3 as a function of time after the inhalation of $^{15}O_2$.

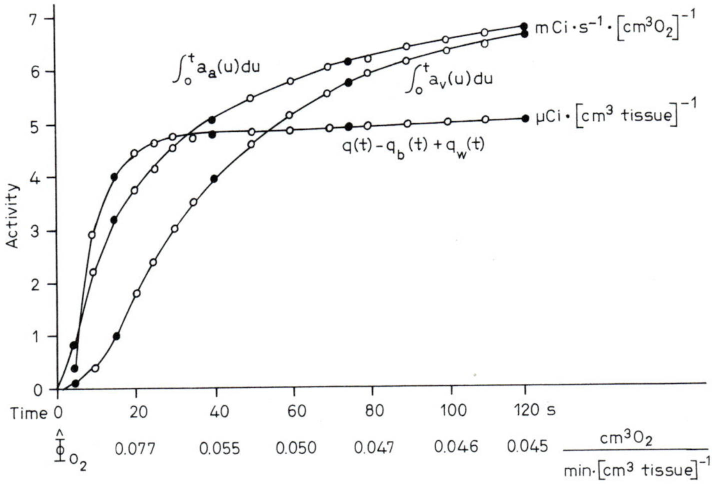

Fig. 3. The time course of the radioactivity in the tissue and of the integral vascular specific activity of oxygen after a bolus inhalation of $^{15}O_2$. q(t) is the total radioactivity per unit weight of brain; $q_b(t)$ is the net loss of radiowater produced in the brain; a_a and a_v are the specific activities of oxygen in carotid and jugular blood.

As the quantities of labeled water metabolically produced in the tissue are known from the stoichiometrical conversion of radioxygen to radiowater, it is possible to tentatively describe the kinetics of water in the brain tissue from these available data by testing in a first step a two-compartment model including only intravascular and extravascular water spaces separated by the blood brain barrier.

If the permeability constant of the brain blood barrier is kept as 0.023 ml s^{-1} g^{-1} [5], estimations can be made for k_{34} and for the apparent values k_{43} and V_3 Figure 2 shows that the apparent extravascular volume of radiowater exceeds 1 ml × [ml tissues]$^{-1}$ and is not stable, especially in the beginning of the production of labeled water. This study therefore gives an approximation of the apparent value of k_{43} and shows that the washout of radiowater should be better described by a three compartmental model (to be published).

(3) The method further allows the definition of criteria for finding the appropriate experimental estimation for the integral in the denominator of equation 12. Figure 3 shows, in a monkey whose CMR_{O_2} is 0.044 ml O_2 min^{-1} [ml tissue]$^{-1}$, that the value obtained for Φ_{O_2} satisfactorily converges toward the independently determined CMR_{O_2}, when the value kept as an estimator of the integral oxygen specific activity in the capillaries is the corresponding arterial integral at its point of convergence with the same integral on the venous side.

These results conclusively show that the arterial specific activity is not a good estimator of the capillary specific activity during the whole time when $^{15}O_2$ exchanges with $^{16}O_2$ in the tissue and that restrictive conditions are to be applied, should the arterial activity be introduced in equation 12 instead of the capillary, inaccessible values.

Beyond this condition of convergence, the results demonstrate that only the arterial specific activity in oxygen is to be considered as the interference of an additional $H_2{}^{15}O$ activity linearly introduced an underestimation of Φ_{O_2}.

The good convergence of the results argues for the feasibility of the measurement of CMR_{O_2} by bolus inhalation of $^{15}O_2$ with a rapid PET detection, using an equation generally formulated as

$$\Phi_{O_2} = \frac{q(t) - q_b(t) + q_w(t)}{\int_0^t a(u)_{O_2}\, du} \qquad (12)$$

where q(t) is the total regional activity in the tissue at time t; $q_b(t)$ is the corresponding activity in the vascular compartment; $q_w(t)$ is the net loss of brain-produced radiowater at time t; a_{O_2} is the specific activity of $^{15}O_2$ – excluding the contribution of $H_2{}^{15}O$ – in the arterial blood the time kept for integration fulfills the convergence condition between integral arterial and venous activities in $^{15}O_2$.

The equation is to be suitably integrated to take into account the duration of collection of data for PET.

The separate determination of $^{15}O_2$ and $H_2{}^{15}O$ activities in the blood also leads to the possibility of actualizing the measurement of the cerebral regional extraction fraction of oxygen from the PET data collected during a continuous inhalation of $^{15}O_2$. In point of fact for the equation deriving this parameter involves the values of $^{15}O_2$ and $H_2{}^{15}O$ activities in the arterial blood during inhalation of $^{15}O_2$ and of $C^{15}O_2$ [11]. Further, the present method offers the opportunity of making sure that the state of equilibrium is effectively reached at the time PET is performed.

Conclusion

The disposal of a method yielding separate determinations of the $^{15}O_2$ and $H_2{}^{15}O$ respective contributions in the blood activity appears to be of importance in the approach to the numerical analysis of the external detection data of the brain after inhalation of $^{15}O_2$.

The application of this technique to animal observations demonstrates the feasibility of a method of measurement of CMR_{O_2} based on a compartmental distribution of oxygen in the brain but also shows some limits of validity of the formula derived from such a model: the main points to be considered in this case are: the imperative of measuring the $^{15}O_2$ activity in arterial blood by withdrawing the rapidly raising contribution of $H_2{}^{15}O$; the necessity of integrating the arterial oxygen specific activity during a sufficiently long time to meet the convergence condition (equalization of the time-integrated arterial and venous oxygen specific activities in the region of interest), and the importance of introducing an estimation of the brain-produced radiowater activity which is washed out the region of interest.

References

1 Kety, S.S.; Schmidt, C.F.: The determination of cerebral blood flow in man by the use of nitrous oxide in low concentration. Am. J. Physiol. *143:* 53–66 (1945).

2 Ter-Pogossian, M.M.; Eichling, J.O.; Davis, D.O.; Welch, M.J.: The measure in vivo of regional cerebral oxygen utilization by means of oxyhemoglobin labeled with radioactive oxygen-15. J. clin. Invest. *49:* 381–391 (1970).

3 Altman, P.; Dittmer, S.: Respiration and circulation. Biological handbooks. Fed. Proc. (1971).
4 Raichle, M.E.; Grubb, J.R.; Ter-Pogossian, M.M.: Measurement of brain oxygen utilization with radioactive oxygen-15: experimental verification. J. appl. Physiol. *40:* 638–640 (1976).
5 Eichling, J.O.: Raichle, M.E.; Grubb, R.L.; Ter-Pogossian, M.M.: Evidence of the limitations of water as a freely diffusible tracer in brain of the rhesus monkey. Circulation Res. *35:* 358–364 (1974).
6 Eichling, J.O.; Gado, M.; Grubb, R.L.; Ter-Pogossian, M.M.: O_2 extraction fraction as an index of cerebral function. J. nucl. Med. (in press).
7 Carter, C.C.; Eichling, J.O.; Davis, D.O.; Ter-Pogossian, M.M.: Correlation of regional cerebral blood flow with regional oxygen uptake using ^{15}O method. Neurology, Minneap. *22:* 755–762 (1972).
8 Grubb, R.L.; Ratcheson, R.A.; Raichle, M.E.; Kliefach, A.B.; Gado, M.H.: Regional cerebral blood flow and oxygen utilization in superficial temporal-middle cerebral artery anastomosis patients. An exploration and definition of clinical problems. J. Neurosurg. *50:* 733–741 (1979).
9 Ter-Pogossian, M.M.; Taveras, J.M.; Davis, D.O.; Eichling, J.O.: A study of regional cerebral oxygen supply and utilization by means of radioactive oxygen-15: in Taveras, Fischgold, Dilenge, Recent advances in the study of the circulation, pp. 156–174 (Thomas, Springfield 1969).
10 Jones, T.; Chesler, D.A.; Ter-Pogossian, M.M: The continuous inhalation of oxygen 15 for assessing regional cerebral extraction in the brain of man. Br. J. Radiol. *19:* 339–343 (1976).
11 Subramanyam, R.; Alpert, N.M.; Hoop, B., Jr.; Brownell, L.; Taveras, J.M.: A model for regional cerebral oxygen distribution during continuous inhalation of $^{15}O_2$, $C^{15}O$ and $C^{15}O_2$. J. nucl. Med. *19:* 48–53 (1978).
12 Mullani, N.A.; Ficke, D.C.; Ter-Pogossian, M.M.: Cesium fluoride: a new detector for positron emission tomography. IEEE Trans. bio-med Electron. *27:* 572–575 (1980).
13 Raichle, M.E.; Welch, W.J.; Grubb, R.L.; Higgins, C.S.; Ter-Pogossian, M.M.; Larson, K.B.: Measurement of regional substrate utilization rates by emission tomography. Science *199:* 986–987 (1978).

J.C. Depresseux, National Foundation of Scientific Research, Cyclotron Research Center, University of Liège, Liège (Belgium)

Eur. Neurol. *20:* 215–218 (1981)

Cerebral Oxygen Consumption in the Rat: Pharmacological Stimulation and Suppression, Role of Catecholaminergic Mechanisms

R. Hemmingsen, D.I. Barry

Department of Psychiatry, Rigshospitalet, Copenhagen, Denmark

Key Words. Cerebral oxygen consumption · Cerebral blood flow · Catecholaminergic regulation

Abstract. The relationship between cerebral oxygen consumption ($CMRO_2$), cerebral blood flow and arterial CO_2 tension was investigated during anaesthesia induced by halothane, pentobarbital, ethanol and nitrous oxide. The results obtained with halothane, pentobarbital and ethanol indicate a relationship between central suppressants and CO_2 in decreasing $CMRO_2$. During nitrous oxide anaesthesia, $CMRO_2$ increased with increasing CO_2 tension, an effect which could be prevented by β-adrenergic receptor blockade. This indicates a role of catecholaminergic mechanisms in $CMRO_2$ regulation (as is the case during immobilization stress and ethanol withdrawal), perhaps as a protective measure providing increased energy supply in the central nervous system during conditions of endogenous or exogenous stress.

Introduction

In an accompanying article [*Barry and Hemmingsen,* 1981], we described a method for rapid and repetitive measurement of the cerebral metabolic rate of oxygen consumption ($CMRO_2$) in the rat. The usefulness and applicability of this method will now be illustrated by some of our studies on pharmacological stimulation and suppression of $CMRO_2$, with particular reference to the role of catecholaminergic mechanisms.

Material and Methods

$CMRO_2$ was studied in male Wistar rats by the method described by *Barry and Hemmingsen* [1981], whereby cerebral blood flow (CBF) is measured by the intra-arterial ^{133}Xe technique for rats [*Hertz* et al., 1977] and $CMRO_2$ is determined from the product of CBF and the arteriovenous (sagittal sinus) difference in blood oxygen content. In all experiments, mean arterial pressure (MAP), arterial CO_2 and O_2 tension ($PaCO_2$, PaO_2) and rectal temperature were monitored and maintained within normal physiological limits unless altered for experimental purposes.

The central nervous system (CNS) suppressants

studied were nitrous oxide (N_2O), halothane, pentobarbital and ethanol; these anaesthetics were administered as follows: *N_2O:* 70% N_2O:30% O_2; animals immobilized with succinyl choline: 20 mg/kg. *Halothane:* 0.8% halothane in 70% N_2O:30% O_2. *Pentobarbital:* 45 mg/kg i.p. and ventilation with 70% N_2O:30% O_2. *Ethanol:* 7–9 g ethanol/kg given by intragastric intubation with a 20% w/v ethanol solution; ventilation with 70% N_2O:30% O_2. All animals were able to breathe spontaneously when taken off the respiration pump (with the exception of the immobilized N_2O group). All groups were studied both during normocapnia ($PaCO_2$ ~ 35–38 mm Hg) and hypercapnia ($PaCO_2$ ~ 80–90 mm Hg – addition of CO_2 to inhaled gas mixture); approximately half of the animals in each group were studied first during normocapnia, the rest were studied first during hypercapnia. In order to investigate if catecholaminergic activity was involved in the $CMRO_2$-CBF response during hypercapnia, the β-adrenergic receptor blocker propranolol (2 mg/kg i.v.) was administered to two groups of N_2O anaesthetized rats, either prior to or following induction of hypercapnia [*Hemmingsen* et al., 1979b]. Statistical differences within groups were tested with Wilcoxon's test for paired data whereas comparison between groups were made by means of Mann-Whitney's test for unpaired data. Correlations were tested by the Spearman test.

Results

The results in the four groups receiving CNS suppressants during normocapnia and hypercapnia are shown in figures 1 and 2, respectively. The normocapnic $CMRO_2$ and CBF in the ethanol group were lower than in the N_2O group ($p < 0.05$), whereas there were no significant differences between the N_2O, halothane and pentobarbital groups. During hypercapnia, $CMRO_2$ tended to be lower than normocapnic values in the pentobarbital ($p < 0.10$), ethanol ($p < 0.05$) and halothane groups (n.s.), whereas $CMRO_2$ tended to be higher during hypercapnia in the N_2O group. The CBF response to induced hypercapnia differed considerably between the groups as indicated in figure 3. When propranolol was administered during hypercapnia (in the N_2O groups), $CMRO_2$ decreased to the normocapnic level and CBF was significantly reduced, although it was still 170% higher than during normocapnia. Propranolol administration during normocapnia (in the N_2O group) reduced $CMRO_2$ to below resting level, blocked the $CMRO_2$ increase during hypercapnia and reduced the CBF response to hypercapnia (fig. 4).

Discussion

The reduced $CMRO_2$ and CBF in the ethanol group indicates a more pronounced CNS suppression than in the other groups: the CBF reduction was probably secondary to reduced metabolism (metabolic CBF regulation) as although MAP was lower (≈ 100 mm Hg) in the ethanol group, rats autoregulate CBF well below this pressure [*Hernandez* et al., 1978]. *Fujishima* et al. [1971] suggested a relationship between normocapnic $CMRO_2$ and CBF response to hypercapnia, and in the ethanol group, which had a low normocapnic $CMRO_2$, the CO_2 reactivity was only 20% of the control value (the N_2O group). However, when all groups were considered together no correlation existed between normocapnic $CMRO_2$ and the reactivity, whereas there was a statistically significant correlation between CO_2 response and *changes* in $CMRO_2$ upon induction of hypercapnia ($p < 0.01$), suggesting a relationship between central depressants and CO_2 in affecting $CMRO_2$. As CO_2 has both CNS-excitatory and CNS-suppressing properties [*Woodbury and Karber,* 1960], the difference in $CMRO_2$ response to hypercapnia during N_2O analgesia and during general anaesthesia may be because the threshold

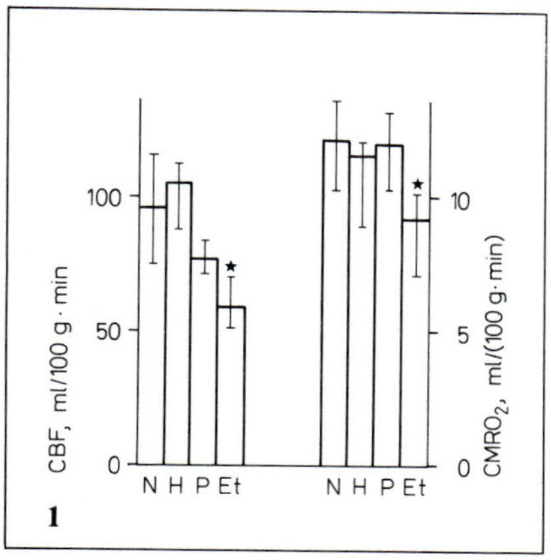

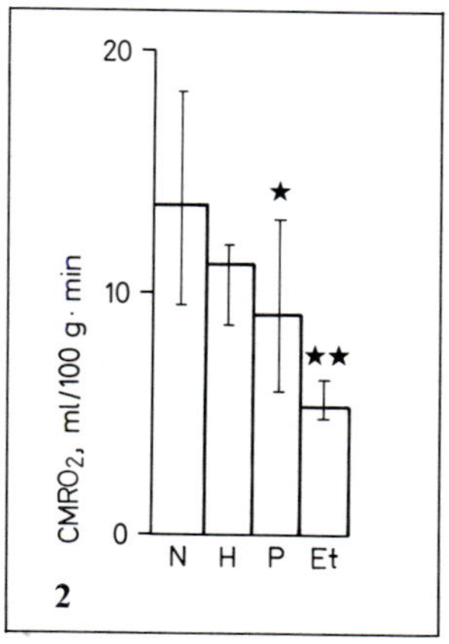

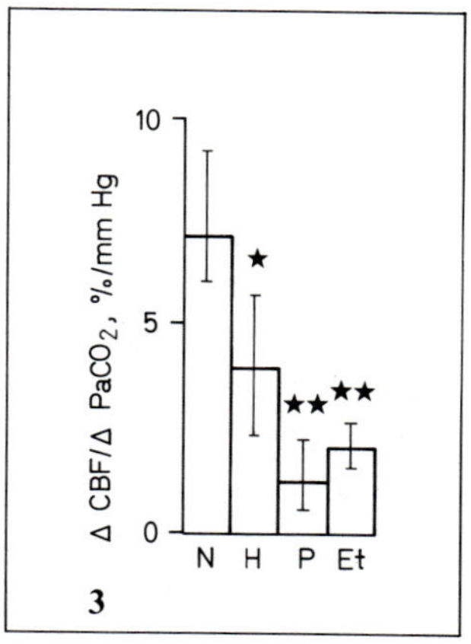

Fig. 1. Cerebral blood flow (CBF) and cerebral oxygen consumption ($CMRO_2$) during normocapnia in animals anaesthetized by nitrous oxide (N; n = 19), halothane (H; n= 8), pentobarbital (P; n = 9) and ethanol (Et; n = 6). Medians and quartiles are indicated. ★ = $p < 0.05$. Comparison with group N.

Fig. 2. $CMRO_2$ during hypercapnia in the same groups as in figure 1. Medians and quartiles are indicated. ★ = $p < 0.10$; ★★ = $p < 0.05$. Comparison with normocapnic values.

Fig. 3. Cerebrovascular reactivity to carbon dioxide expressed in relative terms (percent CBF change per mm Hg increase in $PaCO_2$) in the same groups as in figure 1. Medians and quartiles are indicated. ★ = $p < 0.05$; ★★ = $p < 0.01$. Comparison with nitrous oxide group.

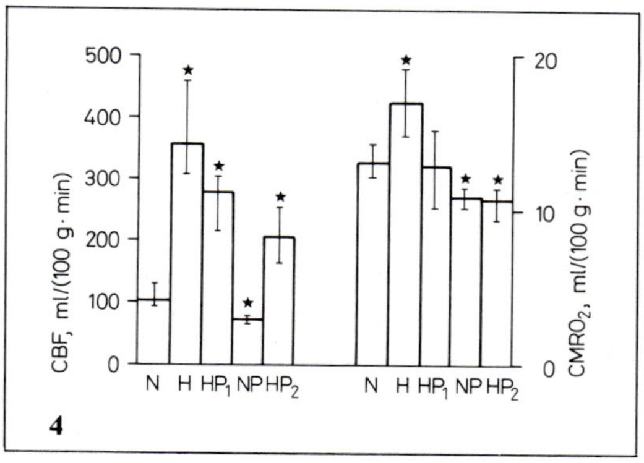

Fig. 4. $CMRO_2$ and CBF during normocapnia and hypercapnia, before and after administration of propranolol (2 mg/kg i.v.) in rats anaesthetized with nitrous oxide. N = Normocapnic controls (n = 7), H = hypercapnic controls (n = 7), HP_1 = propranolol given during hypercapnia (n = 7), NP = normocapnic animals given propranolol (n = 6), HP_2 = propranolol given before induced hypercapnia (n = 6). Medians and quartiles are indicated. ★ = $p < 0.05$ when compared to normocapnic controls.

for the suppressing effect may be lowered by anaesthetics.

The reduction of normocapnic $CMRO_2$ by propranolol supports a previous study in baboons by *MacKenzie* et al. [1976]. Our finding of an increase in $CMRO_2$ during hypercapnia, and that this could be blocked by propranolol, is in good agreement with a similar study by *Berntman* et al. [1979], also in rats. Furthermore, they demonstrate that the $CMRO_2$ response to CO_2 was not blocked by adrenalectomy, indicating that central catecholaminergic mechanisms may be involved in the response. Thus the CBF response during hypercapnia may be the result of two additive mechanisms: (1) a catecholaminergic cerebral activation leading to increased $CMRO_2$ and resultant CBF increase (metabolic regulation), and (2) a direct vascular CO_2 effect (vascular regulation).

The increased O_2 consumption in the brain during hypercapnia is not accompanied by increased glucose consumption: *Miller* et al. [1975] demonstrated that after 5 min of 20% CO_2 inhalation in rats $CMRO_2$ increased whilst CMRgl decreased. The events resulting in the abnormal proportion of O_2 and glucose consumption probably involve a reduced glycolytic rate (the effect of acidosis on the PFK step (PFK = phosphofructokinase). Hypercapnia is not accompanied by changed adenine nucleotide concentration (energy charge), indicating that endogenous substrate (e.g. amino acids) is oxidized in order to maintain energy production [review of metabolic studies, see *Siesjö,* 1978]. Finally, a possible role of uncoupled oxidative phosphorylation cannot be ruled out [*Siesjö,* 1978].

The present study supports the concept of coupling between $CMRO_2$ and cerebrovascular reactivity and indicates that central catecholaminergic mechanisms may be involved. Catecholaminergic involvement in $CMRO_2$ regulation has also been demonstrated during normal conditions [*MacKenzie* et al., 1976], immobilization stress [*Carlsson* et al., 1977] and during ethanol withdrawal [*Hemmingsen* et al., 1979a]. In conclusion, the catecholamines may be considered elements of a neurophysiological regulatory system which continuously influences neuronal level of activity (in turn influencing cerebral vascular state of function – CBF) and which may be a protective measure providing increased energy supply in the CNS during conditions of endogenous or exogenous stress.

References

Berntman, L.; Dahlgren, N.; Siesjö, B.K.: Cerebral blood flow and oxygen consumption in the rat brain during extreme hypercapnia. Anesthesiology *50:* 299–305 (1979).

Carlsson, C.; Hägerdal, M.; Kaasik, A.E.; Siesjö, B.K.: Acatecholamine mediated increase in cerebral oxygen uptake during immobilization stress in rats. Brain Res. *119:* 223–231 (1977).

Fujishima, M.; Sheinberg, P.; Busto, R.; Reinmuth, O.M.: The relationship between cerebral oxygen consumption and cerebral vascular reactivity to carbon dioxide. Stroke *2:* 251–257 (1971).

Hemmingsen, R.; Barry, D.I.; Hertz, M.M.; Klinken, L.: Cerebral blood flow and oxygen consumption during ethanol withdrawal in the rat. Brain Res. *173:* 259–269 (1979a).

Hemmingsen, R.; Hertz, M.M.; Barry, D.I.: The effect of propranolol on cerebral oxygen consumption and blood flow in the rat: measurements during normocapnia and hypercapnia. Acta physiol. scand. *105:* 274–281 (1979b).

Hernandez, M.J.; Brennan, R.W.; Bowman, G.S.: Cerebral blood flow autoregulation in the rat. Stroke *9:* 150–155 (1978).

Hertz, M.M.; Hemmingsen, R.; Bolwig, T.G.: Rapid and repetitive measurements of blood flow and oxygen consumption in the rat brain using intra-arterial xenon injection. Acta physiol. scand. *101:* 501–503 (1977).

MacKenzie, E.T.; McCulloch, J.; Harper, A.M.: Influence of endogenous norepinephrine on cerebral blood flow and metabolism. Am. J. Physiol. *231:* 489–494 (1976).

Miller, A.L.; Hawkins, R.A.; Veech, R.L.: Decreased rate of glucose utilisation by rat brain in vivo after exposure to atmospheres containing high concentrations of CO_2. J. Neurochem. *25:* 553–558 (1975).

Siesjö, B.K.: Brain energy metabolism (Wiley, New York 1978).

Woodbury, D.M.; Karber, R.: The role of carbon dioxide in the nervous system. Anesthesiology *21:* 686–703 (1960).

Dr. Ralf Hemmingsen, Department of Psychiatry, Rigshospitalet, 9 Blegdamsvej, DK–2100 Copenhagen (Denmark)

Eur. Neurol. *20:* 219–220 (1981)

Cerebral Oxygen Consumption and Glucose Consumption during Status epilepticus[1]

Martin Ingvar, Bo K. Siesjö

Laboratory of Experimental Brain Research, University of Lund, Sweden

Key Words. Deoxyglucose · Seizure · CMR_{O_2}, CMR_{gl}, CBF

Abstract. The ^{14}C-deoxyglucose technique has provided us with an extremely valuable technique for functional mapping in different epileptic models. In non-steady-state situations, however, measurements of cerebral oxygen consumption represent the only techniques available for assessment of the metabolic rate.

Cerebral energy consumption is known to be elevated during epileptic seizures. Data on whole brain and cortical oxygen consumption during seizures induced with the GABA-receptor blocker, bicuculline, were published by *Meldrum and Nilsson* [1976]. The method used was a modified *Kety and Schmidt* [1948] technique with sampling of cerebral venous blood from either the sagittal sinus or the retroglenoid vein. With both methods, the results showed an increase in oxygen consumption at 20 min to 250–300% of control. Recently, we have carried out studies using the ^{14}C-deoxyglucose technique of *Sokoloff* et al. [1977] in the same animal model [*Ingvar and Siesjö,* in press]. Since the model yields a sustained seizure activity it lends itself to studies with this technique. The results for cortical structures indicate an increase in metabolic rate for glucose after 20 min to 1 h of seizure activity to approximately 265% of control. The results are thus very much in agreement with those previously mentioned.

Studies of the metabolic rate for oxygen during convulsions due to an acute overdose of the local anesthetic, lidocaine, have been carried out by *Sakabe* et al. [1974]. Dogs infused with lidocaine until seizures occurred were used as models. The authors found a biphasic reaction to the infusion of lidocaine. With increasing doses, CMR_{O_2} fell progressively down to 60% of control. When seizures appeared on the EEG, CMR_{O_2} increased to a mean value of 112% of control. This

[1] Most of the work mentioned in this article was supported by grants from the Swedish Medical Research Council and from NIH.

value is indeed lower than that obtained during status epilepticus induced by bicuculline. A study made by *Ingvar and Shapiro* [in press] in rats may offer an explanation for their finding. Employing the ^{14}C-deoxyglucose technique of *Sokoloff* et al. [1977] we determined the glucose consumption in rats which had received an acute overdose of lidocaine leading to convulsions (20 mg/kg). In almost all structures the metabolic rate was decreased to 50–60% of control, but in the hippocampus-amygdala system there was an increase, and in the hippocampus the average increase was to 240% of control.

The results quoted demonstrate the advantages of both CMR_{O_2} and CMR_{gl} measurements for estimating metabolic demands in the brain during epileptic seizures. Measurements of CMR_{O_2} have a much better time resolution, especially when they are performed with a venous outflow technique for measuring CBF such as that of *Meldrum and Nilsson* [1976]. In some metabolic states, e.g. during short-lasting epileptic activity or other non-steady-state conditions, the deoxyglucose technique cannot be used without extensive corrections. In these conditions the measurement of CBF and oxygen consumption seems superior, provided that it is accepted that information on regional values is not obtained.

The ^{14}C-deoxyglucose technique, on the other hand, yields quantitative estimates of the metabolic rate at the local level, information which is mandatory for an understanding of metabolic correlates to aberrant functional activity. For example, the seemingly paradoxical stability of metabolic rate during lidocaine seizures, as revealed by CMR_{O_2} measurements, receives its explanation when the ^{14}C-deoxyglucose measurements demonstrate that the increase in metabolic rate is almost solely confined to the hippocampus.

References

Ingvar, M.; Shapiro, H.M.: Selective metabolic activation of hippocampus during lidocaine caused preseizure activity. Anesthesiology (in press).

Kety, S.S.; Schmidt, C.F.: The nitrous oxide method for the qualitative determination of cerebral blood flow in man: theory, procedure and normal values. J. clin. Invest. *27:* 476–483 (1948).

Meldrum, B.; Nilsson, B.: Cerebral blood flow and metabolic rate early and late in prolonged epileptic seizures induced in rats by bicuculline. Brain *99:* 523–542 (1976).

Sakabe, T.; Maekawa, T.; Ishikawa, T.; Takeshita, H.: The effects of lidocaine on canine cerebral metabolism and circulation related to the electroencephalogram. Anesthesiology *40:* 433–441 (1974).

Sokoloff, L.; Reivich, M.; Kennedy, C.; Des Rosiers, M.H.; Patlak, C.; Pettigrew, K.; Sakurada, O.; Shinohara, M.: The ^{14}C-deoxyglucose method for the measurement of local cerebral glucose utilization. J. Neurochem. *28:* 897–916 (1977).

Martin Ingvar, Laboratory of Experimental Brain Research, University Hospital,
S–221 85 Lund (Sweden)

Eur. Neurol. *20:* 221–224 (1981)

Inhibition of Cerebral Metabolism by Lidocaine

J. Astrup, H. Rahbek Sørensen

Department of Thoracic and Cardiac Surgery, Rigshospitalet, Copenhagen, Denmark

Key Words. Lidocaine · Cerebral metabolism · Local anesthetics · Barbiturates · Hypothermia · Protection

Abstract. The effects of lidocaine in high doses, i.e. higher than seizure doses, on cerebral function and metabolism are reviewed. Evidence is presented that lidocaine (160 mg/kg) reduces membrane Na^+-K^+ permeability, restricts leak fluxes of these ions, and decreases the load on the associated ion transport. In the ischemic brain (circulatory arrest in dogs on cardiopulmonary bypass circulation), lidocaine delays K^+ efflux, indicating reduced membrane permeability. In the nonischemic brain lidocaine has two effects. One is to abolish electrocortical activity and reduce oxygen and glucose consumption accordingly ('barbiturate-like' effect). The other is a specific membrane sealing effect by which Na^+-K^+ leak fluxes are restricted and associated demand for active transport accordingly reduced. By this effect lidocaine is able to reduce cerebral metabolism by an additional 15–20% below the barbiturate minimum at flat EEG. These effects of lidocaine resemble those of hypothermia and may enhance the hypothermic protection of the ischemic brain.

Introduction

Based on recent studies [1, 2], the effects of a high dose of lidocaine on cerebral function and metabolism are reviewed. The ultimate purpose of these studies has been to gain insight into the cellular work and energy expenditure in the brain, and by specific inhibition of energy-requiring processes (synaptic transmission, Na^+-K^+ leak fluxes and associated transport) to obtain very low levels of cerebral oxygen and glucose consumption. Lidocaine was chosen for study due to its local anesthetic action and its ability to penetrate the blood-brain barrier. Local anesthetics abolish excitation by blocking the associated opening of the Na^+ channels in the membrane [8]. This membrane-sealing effect of lidocaine on peripheral nerves contrasts its seizure-eliciting effect in the brain. In waking monkeys the seizure dose of lidocaine is 20–25 mg/kg [5]. As studied in dogs, lidocaine seizures are associated with metabolic stimulation [7]. Previous studies have concentrated on this seizure-eliciting effect, and higher doses of lidocaine have not been studied. Presumably, the Na^+ channel blocking effect will dominate also in brain at high lidocaine concentrations. Such an action will not only abolish spontaneous synaptic transmission and induce flat EEG, but may also block the Na^+-K^+ fluxes independent of synaptic transmission, i.e. the Na^+-K^+ leak fluxes. This two-sided action of lidocaine in high doses was recently evidenced and correlated to cerebral oxygen and glucose consumption rates ($CMRO_2$ and CMRgluc) [1, 2]. The results show that it is possible by lidocaine to reduce cerebral metabolism below the hitherto described barbiturate minimum obtained at flat EEG [4].

Methods and Results

Dogs on cardiopulmonary bypass circulation were studied. Anesthesia was induced by thiopental and maintained on halothane 1–1.5%. Lidocaine (160 mg/kg) was given as a bolus or as constant rate infusion following barbiturate. This way seizures were avoided. The effect of lidocaine was compared to barbiturate (40 mg/kg thiopental or 40 mg/kg pentobarbital) given either as bolus or infusion. The effects of lidocaine and barbiturate were studied at brain temperature of 37, 28 and 18 °C measured by an inserted thermistor. Epidural chlorinated silver wires monitored EEG. Blood pressure, central venous pressure, hemoglobin concentration, and blood gases were monitored.

Effect of Lidocaine on EEG and Na^+-K^+ Leak Fluxes

160 mg/kg lidocaine given as bolus in the heart-lung machine caused flat EEG within seconds without intermediate signs of spike activity. Barbiturate-induced flat EEG remained flat during lidocaine infusion. It was concluded that spontaneous electrocortical activity is abolished by lidocaine. Barbiturates have a similar action [2, 6] and we may speak of a 'barbiturate-like' effect of lidocaine on brain function (at high doses only).

The effect of lidocaine on Na^+-K^+ leak fluxes were studied during complete cerebral ischemia. Circulatory arrest was obtained by stopping the bypass circulation. In the ischemic brain the Na^+-K^+ ion pump fails due to energy depletion. Na^+ leaks into and K^+ out of the cellular compartment passively following the electrochemical gradient and membrane permeability. The potassium concentration on the brain surface $(K^+)_s$ [which corresponds well to the true extracellular potassium concentration $(K^+)_e$ in the cortex as measured by inserted microelectrodes] was monitored by a potassium selective membrane electrode [1]. Lidocaine delayed and slowed the ischemic $(K^+)_s$ increase indicating reduced Na^+-K^+ exchange leak fluxes. It is reasonable to explain this effect as a Na^+ channel block in analogy to the membrane effect on peripheral nerves. At 37 and 28 °C the $(K^+)_s$ increase rate was reduced by about 30%, at 18 °C by somewhat less. Hypothermia by itself delayed the $(K^+)_s$ increase indicating sealed membranes in cold ischemia. The lidocaine effect was additive to the effect of hypothermia. Thiopental (40 mg/kg) had no effect on the ischemic K^+ efflux indicating no membrane-sealing effect of this drug.

On the basis of these results it was assumed that lidocaine inhibits cerebral metabolism by two different mechanisms. One is the 'barbiturate-like' effect related to the arrest of synaptic transmission. The other is the specific effect related to membrane sealing and reduction of ion transport demand. The metabolic study was designed to show both effects.

Effect of Lidocaine on $CMRO_2$ and CMRgluc

The effect of lidocaine on $CMRO_2$ and CMRgluc was studied in two series: 160 mg/kg lidocaine given as a bolus in the heart-lung machine, and 160 mg/kg lidocaine given as infusion following 40 mg/kg pentobarbital. The first series was included to get the overall effect of lidocaine, i.e. the 'barbiturate-like' effect on synaptic transmission *and* the specific Na^+-K^+ leak flux blocking effect. The second series was included to get the specific Na^+-K^+ leak flux blocking effect *only*. In this series lidocaine acted on the barbiturate EEG arrested brain. Studies were made at brain temperatures of 37, 28 and 18 °C. We used the sagittal sinus outflow method [3, 6]. This method allows continuous measurements of oxygen and glucose consumption in the drained part of the brain. Precautions must be taken to ensure that a constant part of the brain is drained. This is attempted by closing alternative venous outflow routes. Measurements of venous outflow and arteriovenous differences of oxygen and glucose were performed at 5-min intervals.

160 mg/kg lidocaine reduced $CMRO_2$ and CMRgluc by 34.9 ± 4.7 and 38.8 ± 5.1% ($\bar{x}$ ± SEM, n = 6) respectively, using 1% halothane anesthesia as control condition. This is the overall effect of lidocaine. For comparison, 40 mg/kg pentobarbital reduced $CMRO_2$ and CMRgluc by 30.6 ± 5.5 and 25.8 ± 6.1% ($\bar{x}$ ± SEM, n = 6) respectively. These results were obtained at 37 °C. Similar relative reductions in cerebral metabolism were obtained at 28 (n = 3) and 18 °C (n = 3). Following 40 mg/kg pentobarbital, 160 mg/kg lidocaine reduced $CMRO_2$ and CMRgluc by an additional 15.2 ± 3.4 and 19.0 ± 5.3% ($\bar{x}$ ± SEM, n = 6), respectively. This is the specific effect of lidocaine, interpreted as a block of the Na^+-K^+ leak fluxes and associated oxygen and glucose consuming active transport. For comparison, 40 mg/kg pentobarbital given after lidocaine (160 mg/kg) had no effect on metabolism. These results suggest that barbiturates inhibit metabolism by blocking synaptic transmission only, while lidocaine inhibits metabolism *both* by blocking synaptic transmission *and* by a membrane-sealing effect. Lidocaine reduced $(K^+)_s$ increase rate by 30% but metabolism in the barbiturate-arrested brain with flat EEG by only 15–20%. These results seem divergent, since a 30% reduction in Na^+-K^+ leak fluxes is likely to correspond to a similar reduction in transport demand. However, the methods imply such divergence. The Na^+-K^+ transport may well be cut by 30% by lidocaine, but when this effect is measured as metabolic inhibition, it is measured in relation to the total residual oxygen and glucose consumption of which it can only be a fraction smaller than 30%. This leaves part of the residual metabolism in the EEG-arrested brain to hitherto unidentified processes.

Concluding Remarks

Until now, lidocaine is the only drug studied which can reduce cerebral metabolism below the barbiturate minimum obtained at flat EEG. This effect is probably caused by the specific membrane-sealing effect of this local anesthetic drug. Hitherto, hypothermia was the only condition by which cerebral metabolism could be reduced below the barbiturate minimum. Also hypothermia has a membrane-sealing effect as evidenced by the reduced K^+ efflux rates in the ischemic brain at 28 and 18 °C. Thus, the effect of lidocaine resembles that of hypothermia, and the effects are additive. The effects seem specific for lidocaine, while hypothermia inhibits other processes as well. The 'hypothermia-like' effect of lidocaine may therefore not necessarily indicate that lidocaine – as hypothermia – has a protective effect in cerebral ischemia. But this possibility has been proposed [1, 2] and deserves further investigation.

References

1 Astrup, J.; Skovsted, P.; Gjerris, F.; Rahbek Sørensen, H.: Increase in extracellular potassium in the brain during circulatory arrest: effects of hypothermia, lidocaine, thiopental, and hypercapnia. Anesthesiology (submitted).

2 Astrup, J.; Møller Sørensen, P.; Rahbek Sørensen, H.: Inhibition of cerebral oxygen and glucose consumption in the dog by hypothermia, pentobarbital, and lidocaine. Anesthesiology (submitted).

3 Michenfelder, J.D.; Messick, J.M.; Theye, R.A.: Simultaneous cerebral blood flow measured by direct and indirect methods. J. surg. Res. *8:* 475–481 (1968).

4 Michenfelder, J.D.: The interdependency of cerebral function and metabolic effects following massive doses of thiopental in the dog. Anesthesiology *41:* 231–236 (1974).

5 Munson, E.S.; Tucker, W.K.; Ansinsch, B.; Malagodi, M.H.: Etidocaine, bupivacaine, and lidocaine seizure. Thresholds in monkeys. Anesthesiology *42:* 471–478 (1975).

6 Rapela, C.E.; Green, H.D.; Demison, A.B.: Baroreceptor reflexes and autoregulation of cerebral blood flow in the dog. Circulation Res. *21:* 559–568 (1967).

7 Sakabe, T.; Maekawa, T.; Ishikawa, T.; Takeshita, H.: The effect of lidocaine on canine cerebral metabolism and circulation related to the electroencephalogram. Anesthesiology *40:* 433–441 (1974).

8 Strichartz, G.: Molecular mechanism of nerve block by local anesthetics. Anesthesiology *45:* 421–441 (1976).

J. Astrup, MD, Fredensvej 17,
DK–2920 Charlottenlund (Denmark)

Eur. Neurol. *20:* 225–229 (1981)

Continuous Estimation of Cerebral Metabolic Changes

Elisabeth Pinard, Jacques Seylaz

Laboratoire de physiologie cérébrovasculaire, CHU Lariboisière-St.-Louis, Paris, France

Key Words. Mass spectrometry · Cerebral blood flow · Cerebral metabolism · Cerebral PO_2 · Cerebral PCO_2

Abstract. The purpose of the present research has been to estimate rapid metabolic changes. By means of mass spectrometry, the partial pressures of physiological gases are continuously analyzed in a local area of the brain tissue. The method we have developed allows quantitative measurement of the variables with a response time of less than 1 min. When coupled with continuous measurement of (1) PaO_2 and $PaCO_2$ by means of mass spectrometry, and (2) cerebral blood flow by thermoclearance, this method is able to indicate rapid metabolic changes when quantitative methods of determining metabolism are not usable.

Most of the techniques to measure cerebral metabolism need the stability of metabolic and circulatory variables during several minutes [1, 2]. It is therefore impossible to study rapid or polyphasic changes of cerebral metabolism. We, however, attempted to measure continuously the partial pressures of oxygen and carbon dioxide in the brain (PO_2, PCO_2) which might be considered as an index of cerebral metabolism if cerebral blood flow (CBF) and the partial pressures of the arterial oxygen and carbon dioxide (PaO_2, $PaCO_2$) are monitored.

Previous studies [3, 4] have shown that it is possible to analyze physiological gases in biological media by means of mass spectrometry. The present work describes the results we obtained by adapting this technique to deep brain structures with special care to quantify the measured variables.

Materials and Methods

Details of the technique have been published elsewhere [5]. Basically, the method consists of continuously sampling a minute quantity of gases in the tissue. These gases are introduced by means of a high vacuum system in a quadrupole mass spectrometer, they are ionized and then separated according to their molecular weight. A linear signal is provided directly proportional to the partial pressure of each gas sampled. The success of the method resides essentially in the development of a miniature sampling cannula, so that the sampling rate of gases per unit surface be great enough to sensitize the mass spectrometer, and small enough not to deplete the brain tissue. The cannula developed in our laboratory is made of a stainless steel tube (0.4 mm O.D.) which has two holes (drilled on opposite sides of the tube). The tube is enveloped with a hermetically sealed polyethylene membrane (0.5 mm I.D., 0.7). Because the polyethylene does not touch the tube, the gases are sucked across the entire membrane which increases the total amount of gases which reaches the mass spectrometer while decreasing the quantity of gases sampled per unit surface. Thus, the measurement is quantitative and has a response time of 51 s for O_2 and 45 s for CO_2 at 37 °C. There is a dependence between temperature and response time of about 3 s/°C. We have demonstrated in vitro that the measurement is linear. In addition the stability of the method was proved by long measurement periods (15 h) during which variations did not exceed 2%.

This cannula is implanted chronically and stereotaxically in the chosen structure of the animal's brain, 15 days before the experiment (the time which is required to resorb any edema or inflammation [6]). A fiberglass cover is cemented to the skull to protect the cannula.

To control the arterial values of PO_2 and PCO_2 from which cerebral PO_2 and PCO_2 are dependent, mass spectrometry was also used, but with a different cannula [7]. This cannula is made of a stainless steel tube (0.4 mm O.D.) with three holes drilled on only one side of the cylinder. The tube is covered with a thin silicone membrane; this asymmetrical geometry was combined with the flexibility of the connection to be able to turn the probe in the artery till the pumping zone was in front of the arterial lumen. The response time is 8 s, the measurement is quantitative and there is no temperature dependence. At the beginning of the experiment, the cannula is introduced via an aortic catheter placed in the femoral artery. This catheter also allows the measurement of blood pressure.

Cerebral blood flow is registered in the same structure as PO_2 and PCO_2, by means of a thermoclearance method [8]. Two needle-shaped thermoprobes are implanted chronically and stereotaxically the same day as the sampling cannula. One of the thermoprobes is heated a few tenths of a degree above the tissue temperature; the other, being the reference probe, is used for the measurement of the temperature of the tissue. The difference in temperature between the two probes is maintained constant by heating a coil surrounding the thermosensitive element. It has been demonstrated that the variations of the current necessary to heat the coil are directly proportional to the local CBF changes.

Tests of the Method

Figure 1 represents an example of how the probes function during experiments conducted on rabbits. First, papaverine (2.5 mg/kg) is injected intravenously to observe the consequences of an increase in CBF on the measured variables. Of course, while PaO_2 and $PaCO_2$ did not sufficiently change to explain the increase in PO_2 and the decrease in PCO_2, one can observe that the increase in flow induces an amount of oxygen and an elimination of CO_2.

Second, an inhalation of a mixture of air and 7% CO_2 causes, as expected, an increase in $PaCO_2$, followed by an increase in cerebral PCO_2 which is responsible for a marked vasodilation. This dilation induces a larger amount of O_2, thereby increasing the PO_2.

The inhalation of pure oxygen is also a test which is always used. It causes an increase of PaO_2 which nearly doubles the PO_2 value, while CBF changes are very weak.

These two kinds of test show, as expected, that PO_2 and PCO_2 are dependent not only on the cerebral metabolism, but also on vascular reactions and PaO_2, $PaCO_2$, which makes obvious the interest in measuring all these variables simultaneously, if the aim is to estimate cerebral metabolic variations.

Application of the Method

This method is useful when the control of rapid metabolic changes is required, especially to study the mechanisms involved in the cerebrovascular reactions. Two examples of applications have been chosen to show the interest of this method.

The first one comes from a study whose aim was to define the mechanism of action of

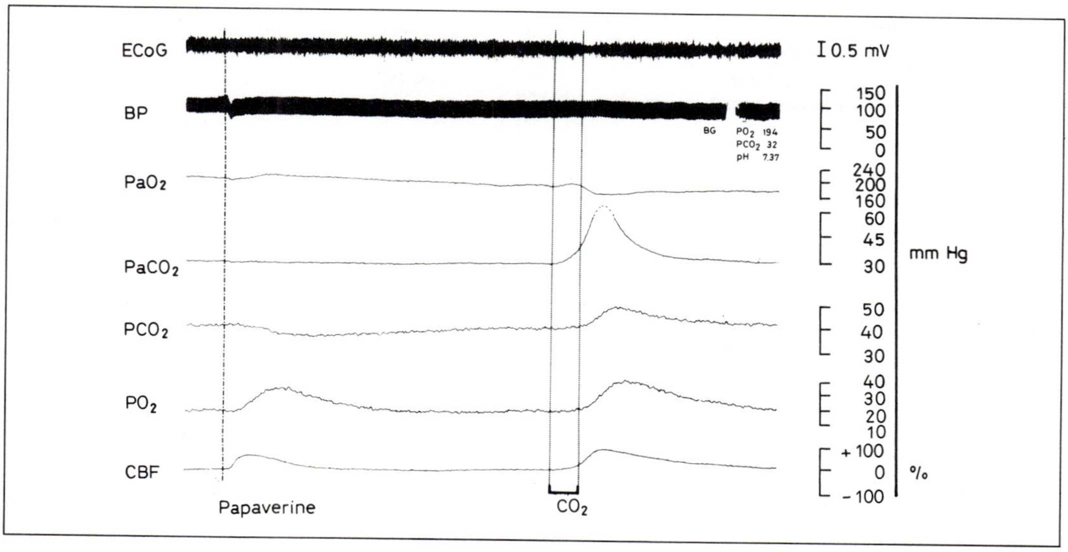

Fig. 1. Effects of an intravenous injection of papaverine (2.5 mg/kg) and of an inhalation of air + 7% CO_2 on the following variables registered on a rabbit. ECoG = Electrocorticogram; BP = aortic blood pressure; PaO_2 = partial pressure of oxygen in aortic blood; $PaCO_2$ = partial pressure of carbon dioxide in aortic blood; PO_2 = partial pressure of oxygen in the caudate nucleus; PCO_2 = partial pressure of carbon dioxide in the caudate nucleus; CBF = blood flow in the caudate nucleus.

catecholamines on cerebral circulation. The question was whether catecholamines act on the cerebral vessel's diameter by a direct stimulation of specific receptors or by means of local PCO_2 changes [9]. 24 rabbits were used for this study, and the results are presented as the mean variation ± SEM expressed as a percentage of the mean baseline value; these results for cerebral variables concern the caudate nucleus. An intravenous injection of adrenaline (1 µg/kg) induces the following changes:

Figure 2 shows one example of this injection: of course, there is an increase in blood pressure which is perhaps responsible for the slight increase in CBF which occurs just before a marked vasoconstriction. This drop in CBF is well confirmed by a decrease in PO_2 and in increase in PCO_2. It is important to note that the method makes obvious the impossibility that PCO_2 can be responsible for the CBF changes since it varies in the opposite direction. This result demonstrates that α-receptors, situated in the walls of cerebral

$\frac{\Delta PO_2}{PO_2} \times 100$	$\frac{\Delta PCO_2}{PCO_2} \times 100$	$\frac{\Delta PaO_2}{PaO_2} \times 100$	$\frac{\Delta PaCO_2}{PaCO_2} \times 100$	$\frac{\Delta BP}{BP} \times 100$
−7.9 ± 3.8	+3.6 ± 1.2	−1.6 ± 2.0	+1.1 ± 1.1	+19.9 ± 3.6

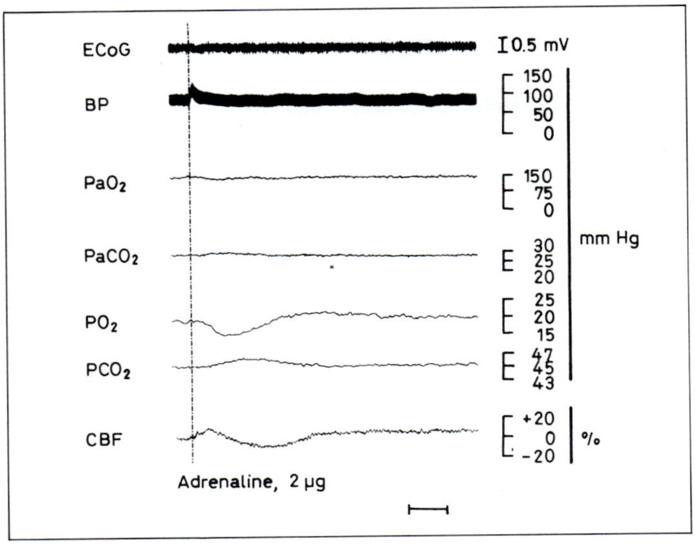

Fig. 2. Effects of an intravenous injection of adrenaline (1 µg/kg) on the same variables as in figure 1.

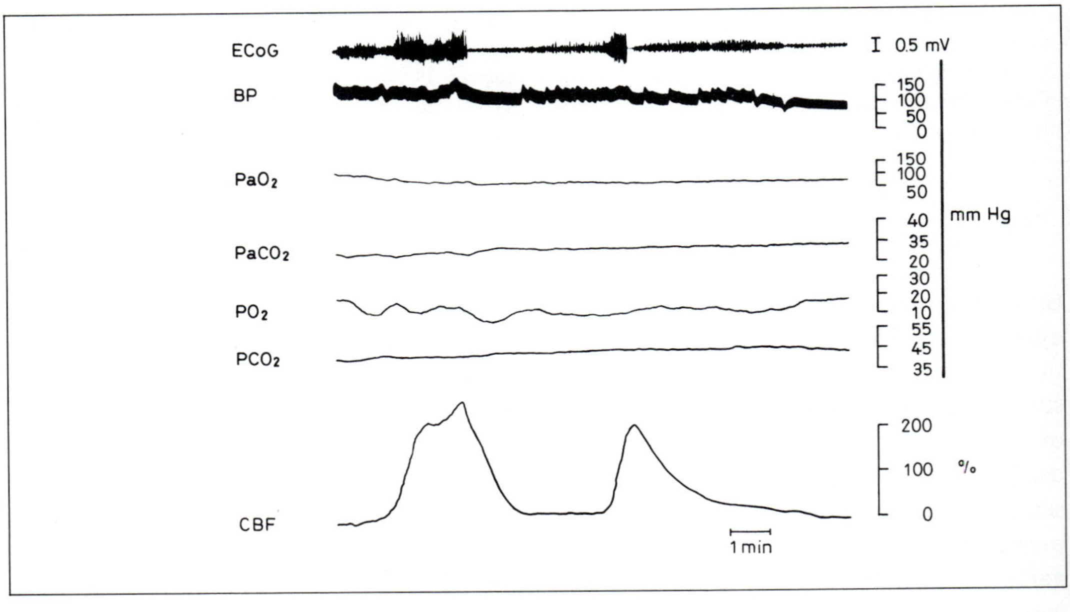

Fig. 3. Effects of an epileptic seizure induced by Megimide (3 mg/kg) on the same variables as in figure 1.

vessels are functional, and that the vascular effects observed are not due to changes of the metabolic variables measured.

The second example of application illustrates preliminary results on epileptic seizures (fig. 3). An enormous increase in flow is contemporary with electrical paroxystic activity, but it is not followed by an increase in PO_2 and a decrease in PCO_2, as expected if only CBF changes had occurred (see tests of the method). This result indicates that the increase in CBF compensates on one hand the consumption of O_2 by a bigger amount of this gas, and on the other hand the production of CO_2 by a greater elimination of this metabolite. In this acute pathological situation CBF changes would be adapted to the metabolic demand of the brain.

Conclusion

Analysis of intracerebral PO_2 and PCO_2 by means of mass spectrometry presents advantages when compared to other techniques. It is continuous, rapid, simultaneous, quantitative, usable on unanesthetized chronically implanted animals. However, to gain a better knowledge of which variables are involved in PO_2 and PCO_2 changes, the method must be combined with simultaneous measurement of CBF and PaO_2 and $PaCO_2$. This method provides an estimation of metabolic variations when rapid cerebral phenomena must be studied, i.e. when quantitative direct methods cannot be applied.

References

1 Sokoloff, L.; Reivich, M.; Patlack, C.S.; Pettigrew, K.D.; des Rosiers, M.; Kennedy, C.: The ^{14}C-deoxyglucose method for the quantitative determination of local cerebral glucose consumption. Trans. Am. Soc. Neurochem. *5:* 85 (1974).

2 Raichle, M.E.; Grubb, R.L., Jr.; Eichling, J.O.; Ter-Pogossian, M.M.: Measurement of brain oxygen utilization with radioactive oxygen-15: experimental verification. J. appl. Physiol. *40:* 638–640 (1976).

3 Woldring, S.; Owens, G.; Woolford, D.C.: Blood gases: continuous in vivo recording of partial pressures by mass spectrography. Science *153:* 885–887 (1966).

4 Roberts, M.; Thomas, D.; Owens, G.; Vilinskas, J.; O'Rourke, J.: A new small diameter mass spectrometer cannula for medical use. Med. Res. Eng. *11:* 27–28 (1972).

5 Seylaz, J.; Pinard, E.: Continuous measurement of gas partial pressures in intracerebral tissue. J. appl. Physiol. *44:* 528–533 (1978).

6 Edvinsson, L.; Nielsen, K.C.; Owman, C.; West, K.A.: Alterations in intracranial pressure, blood brain barriers, and brain oedema after sub-chronic implantation of a cannula into the brain of conscious animals. Acta physiol. scand. *82:* 557–531 (1971).

7 Seylaz, J.; Pinard, E.; Correze, J.L.; Aubineau, P.; Mamo, H.: Continuous measurement of blood gas tensions by mass spectrometry. J. appl. Physiol. *37:* 937–941 (1974).

8 Seylaz, J.: Biophysique de la mesure rapide de l'irrigation sanguine locale. Helv. physiol. pharmacol. Acta *26:* 1–32 (1968).

9 Pinard, E.; Seylaz, J.: Intracerebral gas partial pressure changes under vasoactive drugs. Pflügers Arch. *375:* 25–30 (1978).

Elisabeth Pinard, Laboratoire de Physiologie et Physiopathologie cérébrovasculaire,
10, avenue de Verdun, F–75010 Paris (France)

Eur. Neurol. *20:* 230–234 (1981)

Recovery from Global Cerebral Ischemia in Rabbits: Influence of Indomethacin

R.G. Boulu, C. Gueniau, M. Plotkine, M. Sofeir

Laboratoire de Pharmacodynamie, UER Mécanismes d'action des médicaments et des toxiques, Université René-Descartes, Paris, France

Key Words. Rabbits · Cerebral ischemia · Indomethacin

Abstract. A 10-min cerebral ischemia was induced in rabbits by a combination of vascular occlusion (carotid and vertebral arteries) and systemic hypotension. Cerebral cortex blood flow, cortical pO_2, arterial pH, arterial blood gases, arterial pressure and electrocorticogram were recorded before, during and for 4 h after ischemia. Indomethacin (4 mg · kg^{-1} i.v.) was administered 45 min before or immediately after ischemia. Pretreatment with indomethacin improved cortical reperfusion but did not influence cortical pO_2 and electrocorticographic activity. Post-ischemic treatment did not affect the different measurements. Water and electrolyte contents remained unchanged.

Introduction

There is strong evidence that prostaglandins are implicated in the cerebral blood flow modulation under normal and abnormal conditions [3]. As vasoactive prostaglandins are formed during different types of brain injury including ischemia, it has been hypothesized that the prostaglandin system could be involved in the sequence leading to post-ischemic impairment of microvascular perfusion [4, 5]. Particularly, an imbalance between thromboxane A_2 and prostacyclin might occur. These considerations led *Hallenbeck and Furlow* [5] to investigate the effect of indomethacin, a potent inhibitor of prostaglandin synthesis, on post-ischemic reperfusion in dogs. Improved recirculation was observed only when indomethacin was administered before ischemia [5].

The present study was designed to examine whether the beneficial influence of indomethacin on post-ischemic recirculation is associated with an improved electrocorticographic (ECoG) activity and with a reduction in brain edema.

Materials and Methods

Surgical Preparation

21 male rabbits weighing between 2.1 and 3.7 kg were employed. The animals were curarized (gallamine triethiodide) and ventilated with a mixture of 70% nitrous oxide and 30% oxygen. Arterial CO_2 was maintained between 27 and 32 mm Hg by adjusting the respiratory pump. Before starting surgery, halothane was added to the inhaled gas mixture in a proportion between 0.2 and 0.6%. A 2-cm incision was made bilaterally in the area of the pleural dome to expose vertebral and subclavian arteries. These arteries were ligated permanently. Both carotid arteries were isolated. A catheter was introduced into the aorta through the left femoral artery in order to enable blood pressure recording and to collect blood samples. Needle electrodes were placed into the right foreleg and left hindleg to allow recording of the ECG. A catheter was placed into the left femoral vein for infusion of various solutions. Following completion of the surgical preparation, halothane was stopped and a first dose of heparine (500 $U \cdot kg^{-1}$) was administered intravenously; an additional dose of 250 $U \cdot kg^{-1}$ was given 2 h later.

Physiological Measurements

Cerebral cortex blood flow (CBF) was measured by the hydrogen clearance technique. Hydrogen was added to the inhaled gases (5%). CBF was calculated from the initial slope of the clearance curve [1]. Cortical oxygen tension (pO_2) was measured continuously by the polarographic method and expressed as percentage of the mean pre-ischemic value. ECoG activity was recorded from four derivations (fronto-frontal, occipito-occipital, right fronto-occipital, left fronto-occipital). ECoG, pO_2 and pH_2 electrodes were implanted 2–4 weeks before the experiment. Platinum electrodes (150 μm) were used for pO_2 and pH_2 measurements in frontal cortex. Silver ECoG electrodes were placed on the dura mater. Rectal temperature was kept at 39 °C. Hematocrit was measured with a micromethod. Following a 4-hour recovery period, the rabbits were sacrified by injecting ClK. The water and electrolyte (Na, K) contents of the brains were determined according to *Levine and Torrelio* [7].

Experimental Design

Two measurements of the flow were first taken half an hour after halothane was stopped. Once the control values were obtained, trimetaphan camphosulfonate (50 mg) was infused to allow mean arterial pressure to decrease towards 50–60 mm Hg. Cerebral ischemia was immediately induced by clamping both common carotid arteries and maintained for 10 min. At the end of ischemia, mean pressure was raised to 100–110 mm Hg by infusion of metaraminol (50 μg). CBF was measured during ischemia (after 5 min) and post-ischemic period (5, 30, 60, 120, 180 and 240 min). ECoG, ECG (D II), cortical pO_2 and arterial pressure were recorded continuously.

The animals used were divided into three groups of 7. The rabbits of the first group received 4 $mg \cdot kg^{-1}$ indomethacin (Merck Sharp & Dohme) 45 min prior to ischemia. The drug, dissolved in an aqueous solution of sodium chloride (0.88%) and sodium bicarbonate (0.07%), was infused intravenously. CBF and blood gases were determined 5 min after infusion. In 7 other rabbits, indomethacin was administered at the beginning of recirculation. 7 control animals were given the solvent of indomethacin.

The data from three groups were compared statistically using variance analysis and Student's t test.

Results

The evolution of cerebral blood flow is given in figure 1. It can be seen that only treatment prior to ischemia was capable of improving cortical recirculation. As to cortical pO_2, we observed, in all the three groups, a sharp drop during ischemia, an increase during post-ischemic hyperemia and a return to normal levels 30 min after ischemia. No statistical differences were noted between groups. Table I shows that the times for ECoG flattening and for ECoG reappearance were not influenced by indomethacin given before or after ischemia. Moreover the mean frequency of ECoG was not affected through the recovery period. Table II indicates that brain contents in water and electrolytes (Na, K) 4 h after ischemia were similar among experimental groups.

Arterial pH was slightly decreased during ischemia as well as during post-ischemic hy-

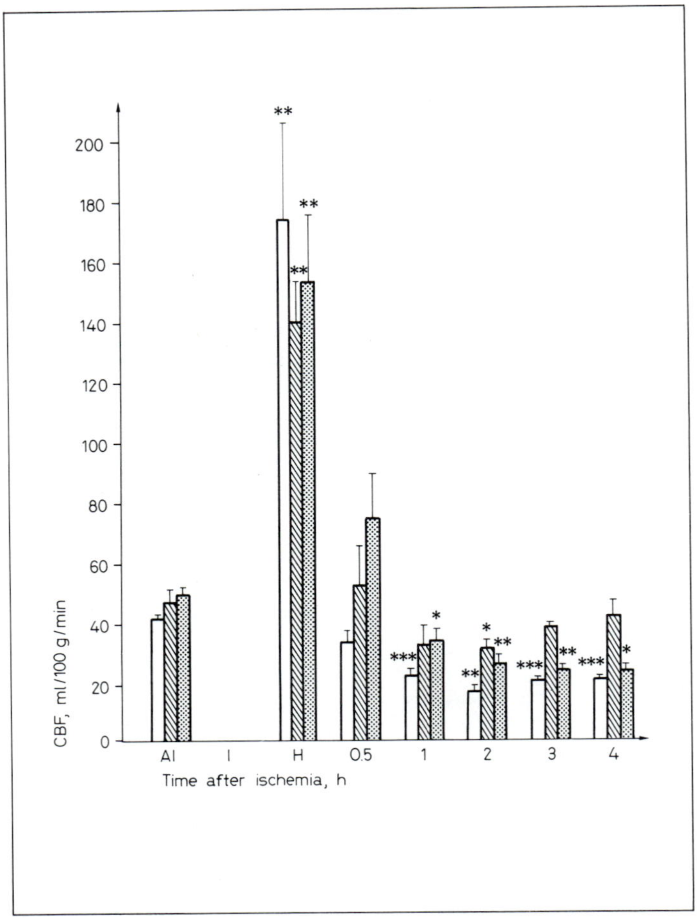

Fig. 1. Evolution of blood flow in the frontal cortex of rabbits submitted to cerebral ischemia (mean ± SEM). AI = Before ischemia; I = ischemia, H = post-ischemic hyperemia. Blank columns = Controls; striped columns = rabbits treated by indomethacin ($4\ mg \cdot kg^{-1}$ i.v.) 45 min prior to ischemia; dotted columns = rabbits treated by indomethacin ($4\ mg \cdot kg^{-1}$ i.v.) after ischemia. * $p < 0.05$; ** $p < 0.01$; *** $p < 0.001$ (comparison with preischemic values). At 3 and 4 h, CBF was higher in rabbits pretreated by indomethacin.

peremia in control rabbits and in rabbits treated with indomethacin after ischemia ($p < 0.001$), but it was maintained at the preischemic level in indomethacin-pretreated animals. The evolution of $paCO_2$ was not significantly influenced by either treatment. A decrease in arterial pO_2 was observed during the 10-min period of ischemia in control animals (108.8 ± 9.1 to 78.1 ± 6.3 mm Hg, $p < 0.05$), but not in pretreated animals. The hypertensive peak recorded in control rabbits during the early phase of post-ischemic recovery (10–30 min) was decreased by indomethacin pretreatment. Hematocrit values were similar among the three groups.

Discussion

The above results are in accordance with previous findings which demonstrated that indomethacin can improve post-ischemic brain reperfusion when given before but not after cerebral ischemia [5]. Our study indi-

Table I. Effect of indomethacin (4 mg · kg^{-1}, i.v.) on ECoG activity in rabbits submitted to 10 min of cerebral ischemia (mean ± SEM)

	No treatment	Indomethacin 45 min before ischemia	Indomethacin immediately after cerebral ischemia
Latency time for ECoG flattening, s	13.4 ± 0.9 (7)	15.5 ± 1.3 (7)	14.0 ± 2.5 (4)
Latency time for ECoG reappearance, min	22 ± 2 (5)	26 ± 4 (7)	26 ± 3 (6)

The figures in parentheses indicate the numbers of animals studied.

Table II. Water and electrolytes in rabbit brains (mean ± SEM)

	No ischemia no treatment I	Ischemia no treatment II	Ischemia indomethacin 4 mg · kg^{-1} before ischemia III	Ischemia indomethacin 4 mg · kg^{-1} after ischemia IV
Water, %	78.5 ± 0.2 (6)	79.2 ± 0.2 (7)*	79.0 ± 0.2 (6)*	79.2 ± 0.1 (6)**
Na, mEq · kg^{-1}, dry weight	260.0 ± 1.7 (5)	277.0 ± 5.9 (7)*	271.3 ± 7.8 (6)	286.5 ± 7.6 (6)*
K, mEq · kg^{-1}, dry weight	425.6 ± 7.5 (5)	433.1 ± 5.0 (7)	439.0 ± 9.1 (6)	438.3 ± 3.5 (6)

The brains were removed 4 h after ischemia. The figures in parentheses indicate the numbers of brains studied.

* $p < 0.05$; ** $p < 0.01$ (comparison with I). No significant differences were observed between II, III and IV.

cates that improved recirculation is accompanied neither by improved ECoG activity nor by reduced post-ischemic brain edema, suggesting that increased blood flow is not sufficient to promote recovery of neuronal function. As indomethacin, a potent inhibitor of prostaglandin synthesis, prevents impairment of post-ischemic reperfusion only when administered before ischemia, it can be suggested that certain prostaglandin compounds formed during ischemia might contribute to the post-ischemic non-reflow phenomenon. There is some experimental evidence that thromboxane A_2 could participate in the process leading to impairment of microvascular perfusion [6]. So it can be expected that drugs which specifically inhibit thromboxane A_2 synthesis would be more efficient than indomethacin in enhancing post-ischemic brain recovery. Moreover, the indomethacin-induced decrease in cerebral blood flow, already observed in baboons [9] and conscious rabbits [2], supports the hypothesis that prostaglandins are involved in the control of CBF. However, it cannot be excluded that indomethacin acts by mechanisms other than inhibition of prostaglandin synthesis [8].

References

1 Auckland, K.; Bower, B.F.; Berliner, R.W.: Measurement of local blood flow with hydrogen gas. Circulation Res. *14:* 164–187 (1964).

2 Bill, A.: Effects of indomethacin on regional blood flow in conscious rabbits – a microsphere study. Acta physiol. scand. *105:* 437–442 (1979).

3 Ellis, E.F.; Wei, E.P.; Kontos, H.A.: Vasodilatation of cat cerebral arterioles by prostaglandins D_2, E_2, G_2 and I_2. Am. J. Physiol. *237:* H381–H385 (1979).

4 Furlow, T.W., Jr.; Hallenbeck, J.M.: Indomethacin prevents impaired perfusion of dog's brain after global ischemia. Stroke *9:* 591–594 (1978).

5 Hallenbeck, J.M.; Furlow, T.W., Jr.: Prostaglandin I_2 and indomethacin prevent impairment of post-ischemic brain reperfusion in the dog. Stroke *10:* 629–637 (1979).

6 Hamberg, M.; Svensson, J.; Samuelsson, B.: Thromboxanes: a new group of biologically active compounds derived from prostaglandin endoperoxides. Proc. natn. Acad. Sci. USA *72:* 2994–2998 (1975).

7 Levine, S.; Torrelio, M.: Cerebral inflammation and edema: a model in rats for testing antiinflammatory drugs. Expl Neurol. *56:* 361–369 (1977).

8 Northover, B.J.: Indomethacin – a calcium antagonist. Gen. Pharmacol. *8:* 293–296 (1977).

9 Pickard, J D.; MacKenzie, E.T.: Inhibition of prostaglandin synthesis and the response of baboon cerebral circulation to carbon dioxide. Nature new Biol. *245:* 187–188 (1973).

R.G. Boulu, PhD, Laboratoire de Pharmacodynamie, UER Mécanismes d'action des médicaments et des toxiques, Université René-Descartes, 4, avenue de l'Observatoire, F–75006 Paris (France)

Eur. Neurol. *20:* 235–244 (1981)

Metabolic Changes Induced by Acute Hypoxia on the Synaptosomes from Dog Brain

G. Benzi, E. Arrigoni, O. Pastoris, S. Raimondo, D. Fulle, D. Curti, R.F. Villa[1]

Department of Science, Institute of Pharmacology, University of Pavia (Italy)

Key Words. Hypoxia · Synaptosomes · Phenobarbital · Papaverine · (–)Eburnamonine

Abstract. Synaptosomal preparations from the motor area of the cerebral cortex of normocapnic, normoxic or hypoxic untreated beagle dogs and phenobarbital-, papaverine-, and (–)eburnamonine-treated dogs were incubated for 10 min at 24 °C and analyzed for ATP, ADP, AMP, creatine phosphate, pyruvate, and lactate. The data were compared with those obtained from the whole controlateral cortical motor area, by the surface-freezing technique. Both during normoxia and after hypoxic hypoxia (15 min, at PaO_2 equal to 17–19 mm Hg) the metabolite contents and ratios were very different in the incubated synaptosomal preparations and in the whole cerebral tissues. As concerns the drug treatment, papaverine was always inactive, while (–)eburnamonine increased the synaptosomal phosphorylation state in hypoxic dogs, being ineffective on the glycolytic metabolites evaluated. Phenobarbital increased the synaptosomal phosphorylation state both in normoxic and in hypoxic animals, and was effective also on the glycolytic metabolites studied.

Introduction

Continuous evaluations of NADH fluorescence from the exposed rat cerebral cortex [*Chance* et al., 1962, 1964; *Chance and Schoener,* 1962] showed no change until the inspired oxygen concentration was reduced below about 8%, in the absence of any significant decrease of NAD^+ until the oxygen concentration was reduced below about 5%. This indicates an efficient O_2 utilization by brain mitochondria. In the same way, during spontaneous ventilation no increase in the cerebral lactate content was observed [*Gurdjian* et al., 1944] until the inspired oxygen concentration was reduced below about 10%, in the absence of any appreciable breaking down of creatine phosphate until the inspired O_2 concentration fell below about 8%.

[1] We thank Mrs. *G. Garlaschi* for technical assistance.

On the other hand, in the rat when the arterial oxygen partial pressure (PaO_2) was reduced below about 50 mm Hg [*Siesjö and Nilsson,* 1971; *MacMillan and Siesjö,* 1971; *Siesjö and Plum,* 1973], there were progressive increases in the intracellular and extracellular lactate concentrations consistent with the observed [*Kogure* et al., 1970] increases in blood flow and in surface acidity. When the PaO_2 was reduced below 35 mm Hg, a relevant increase in lactate and a progressive breaking down of creatine phosphate, without significant changes in the energy charge potential of the adenine nucleotide system was observed [*Siesjö and Nilsson,* 1971; *MacMillan and Siesjö,* 1971]. However, at PaO_2 below about 20 mm Hg, a moderate decrease in the systemic blood pressure induced a severe fall in the energy charge potential [*Benzi* et al., 1978; *Benzi and Villa,* 1976]. The stimulation of glycolysis in spite of both normal energy charge and increased lactacidosis may be slightly related to the increase in the cerebral content of ammonia [*Hindfelt and Siesjö,* 1971], the activation of adenyl cyclase system being more effective [*Benzi and Villa,* 1976].

On the cerebral synapses hypoxia induces modifications in polarization of the neuronal membrane and a failure of neurotransmission [*Grossman and Williams,* 1971; *Silver,* 1973]. In this field, the isolation and preparation of the nerve ending particles or synaptosomes [*Gray and Whittaker,* 1962; *De Robertis* et al., 1962] is indicated [*Rafalowska* et al., 1980a, b] as a suitable model for the characterization of the effects induced by hypoxia and/or pharmacological treatment on the nerve cells. The respiratory rate was decreased in synaptosomal preparations from starved hypoxic rats, but was not significantly different from the respective control values in preparations from hypoxic nembutal-anesthetized animals or from hypoxic non-anesthetized animals allowed to recover from the hypoxic episode by 60 min of normoxic conditions [*Rafalowska* et al., 1980a]. In addition, calculations of the free energy relationships between the mitochondrial redox reactions and ATP synthesis showed that in synaptosomes isolated from the brains of nembutal-anesthetized rats the first two sites of oxidative phosphorylation were at near-equilibrium, in agreement with results from intact cells and tissues [*Rafalowska* et al., 1980b]. Unlike nerve tissue in general, synaptosomes preferentially utilized endogenous ATP and phosphocreatine stores which, on incubation in the absence of exogenous substrates, were emptied long before glycogen stores were exhausted. The synaptosomal respiration rate probably reflects a consumption of the glycogen stores, glucose being devoid of effects on this respiration rate or slightly increasing it [*Jansson* et al., 1979].

The present study shows the effects induced by hypoxia and pharmacological treatment with phenobarbital, papaverine and (–)eburnamonine on some biochemical parameters in suspensions of incubated synaptosomes obtained from the motor area of cerebral cortex of beagle dogs. As concerns the effects induced by hypoxia, in the controlateral area of cerebral cortex the behavior of the same parameters was also evaluated in the whole tissue by the surface-freezing technique.

Methods

Animals and Anesthesia

The experiments were carried out on female beagle dogs aged 1.5 years and weighing from 10.8 to 14.1 kg, maintained under standard environmental conditions (temperature = 22 ± 1 °C; relative humidity = 60 ± 5%) and fed a standard diet as pellets, with water ad libitum.

The surgical procedure was performed on animals starved overnight and preanesthetized with urethane (0.4 g/kg i.p.). Anesthesia was induced and maintained during the surgical procedure by chloralose (40 mg/kg i.v.) and by intermittent nitrous oxide inhalation. During the operative procedure and the experiment, the animals were treated with an intravenous injection of gallamine triethiodide (2–3 mg/kg) to permit unresisted artificial respiration and to maintain a constant $PaCO_2$. The dogs were artificially ventilated with air (normocapnic normoxic condition) or with a 95:5 nitrogen:oxygen mixture (normocapnic hypoxic condition).

The changes in the energy charge of the brain induced by hypoxemia are magnified by the decrease in the arterial blood pressure [*Siesjö and Nilsson,* 1971; *Benzi and Villa,* 1976; *Benzi* et al., 1978]. Therefore the experiments were carried out in hypovolemic hypotension (MABP = 55 ± 4 mm Hg): the dogs were slowly bled within 15 min from an arterial femoral cannula into a heparinized bottle, with three openings to withdraw and oxygenate the blood from systemic circulation. The bottle was connected to a femoral vein to reinfuse (if necessary) the drained blood into the systemic circulation by means of a peristaltic pump.

Operative Procedure

The procedure [*Benzi* et al., 1978] consisted mainly in isolating both common carotid arteries, while the zygomatic, maxillary, auricular, and supraorbital vessels were all occluded by ligature or compression. The head was fixed to a head-holder with the confluence of the cerebral venous sinuses approximately 10 cm higher than the heart. After bilateral longitudinal incisions of skin and muscles, two 2.5–3.5 cm diameter holes were made in the frontal-parietal bones of the skull. A plastic funnel was fitted into each hole and both muscle and skin were sutured tightly around the funnels. These were sealed with a rubber stopper and insulated to prevent untoward ambient heat and pressure exchange.

Both femoral arteries were cannulated: one connected to a physiological pressure transducer and the other to the heparinized bottle to withdraw blood from systemic circulation. Electrical activity of the brain, as portrayed by electroencephalography, was used to determine the degree of anesthesia. Physiological parameters were recorded using a 12-channel recorder (Physioscript EE12, Schwarzer).

Experimental Plan

After the operative procedure, a period of 30 min was allowed before the hypovolemic hypotension was induced. The MABP of 55 mm Hg was attained within 15 min and then cautious arterial withdrawals or venous reinfusions by the peristaltic pump were made so that the mean blood pressure was held as constant as possible from 15 to 30 min. Normally, the blood pressure could be held at the specific level within ± 4.0 mm Hg. If large variations occurred or if a substantial part of the blood had to be reinfused to keep the blood pressure constant, the dog was discarded.

The two experimental periods were: (1) steady-state period of hypovolemic hypotension of 30 min during air ventilation (control condition: PaO_2 102.3 ± 3.3 and $PaCO_2$ 37.1 ± 1.0 Torr); at the end of this steady-state period, cerebral samples for control determinations were obtained (normoxic normocapnic dogs); (2) steady-state period of hypovolemic hypotension of 15 min during air ventilation plus 15 min of acute hypoxia induced in the hypovolemic dogs by altering the inspired oxygen concentration with a 5:95 oxygen:nitrogen mixture in the artificial respirator. Under these conditions PaO_2 ranged between 17 and 19 mm Hg, while $PaCO_2$ ranged between 36 and 39 mm Hg. At the end of this hypoxemic period, cerebral samples for determinations were obtained (hypoxic normocapnic dogs). During both periods 1 and 2, an intracarotid perfusion (into the superior thyroid arteries) at the rate of 0.1 ml · min^{-1} · kg^{-1} was performed (Palmer pump) with: (a) saline solution; (b) phenobarbital, 5×10^{-3} *M;* (c) papaverine, 1×10^{-4} *M;* (d) (–)eburnamonine, 5×10^{-4} *M.*

Withdrawal of Cerebral Samples

At the set time, a portion of the motor area of cerebral cortex was removed from the plastic funnel fitted into one side of the skull. The cortical portion of the cerebral tissue was isolated, and immersed in a cold solution of 0.32 *M* sucrose. The sucrose-washed (0.32 *M)* and weighed tissue was homogenized in 0.32 *M* sucrose for 30 s (precooled Potter-Braun S homogenizer, with a Teflon pestle rotating at 1,000 rpm) for subsequent synaptosomal preparation.

The controlateral portion of the motor area of the brain was frozen in situ by liquid nitrogen and removed from the plastic funnel fitted into the other side of the skull. This portion of the brain was cut in situ by means of a rotating hollow tube, during liquid nitrogen perfusion. The isolated cerebral material was quickly removed by means of a cooled clamp and then immediately immersed into liquid nitrogen for 10–15 min. The cortical portion of the frozen tissue was isolated and quickly (3–4 s) powdered in a precooled automatic apparatus (Microdismembrator, Braun) using frozen 1.23 *M* perchloric acid. The subsequent steps were carried out in a precooled box at 0–5 °C until a neutral perchlorate-free extract was obtained for immediate analyses of metabolites.

Synaptosomal Preparation and Incubation

The diluted (10% w/v) homogenate of the motor area of the cerebral cortex was submitted to fractioning [*De Robertis* et al., 1962] carried out at 0–4 °C, for isolating the crude synaptosomal fraction, obtained as a pellet.

The synaptosomal pellet was washed in Krebs-Henseleit-Hepes (144 m*M* NaCl; 5 m*M* KCl; 5 m*M* $NaHCO_3$; 1.3 m*M* $MgSO_4$; 1 m*M* P_i; 10 m*M* Hepes) pH 7.4 buffer and suspended for the subsequent incubation (about 6–8 mg protein/ml) in this medium plus 10 m*M* glucose and 2 m*M* $CaCl_2$, for 10 min at 24 °C. At the set time, the reactions were stopped by the addition of cold perchloric acid, at 3.5% final concentration. The neutralized extract was then used for immediate metabolite analyses.

Analytical Techniques

The cerebral and synaptosomal extracts were utilized for analyses of: ATP [*Lamprecht and Trautschold,* 1974]; ADP and AMP [*Jaworek* et al., 1974]; creatine phosphate [*Lamprecht* et al., 1974]; pyruvate [*Czok and Lamprecht,* 1974], and lactate [*Gutmann and Wahlefeld,* 1974]. The energy charge potential [*Atkinson,* 1968] was defined in terms of actual concentrations of the adenine nucleotides as: ([ATP] + 0.5[ADP])/([ATP] + [ADP] + [AMP]). The oxygen consumption of the synaptosomal pellets was measured with a Clark-type oxygen electrode at 24 °C in Krebs-Henseleit-Hepes pH 7.4 medium, containing 2 m*M*-$CaCl_2$.

PaO_2 and $PaCO_2$ were measured using anaerobic samples of blood from the carotid arteries (BMS3-Mk2 Blood Micro System, Radiometer).

Measurements of the cytochrome c and a content of synaptosomes were performed as described previously [*Rafalowska* et al., 1980b].

Statistical Analysis

Student's t test or Dunnett's test was applied to the differences in the various instances.

Results

Effect of Hypoxia on Metabolite Content

Table I shows the contents of various metabolites both in whole cerebral tissue from the frozen motor area of the cerebral cortex and in synaptosomes isolated from the controlateral area and incubated at 24 °C for 10 min. The first set of data points out the actual changes induced by hypoxia in the whole tissue, while the second set of data depicts what synaptosomes remember of the hypoxic *noxa* and that cannot be reversed during the further incubation in vitro. In the whole tissue of the motor area of cerebral cortex from the beagle dog in hypovolemic hypotension, hypoxia induced an increase of both lactate (×9.7) and pyruvate (×2.4). Also in the incubated synaptosomal pellets, hypoxia induced an increase of both lactate (× 1.5) and pyruvate (× 1.2), but the magnification was much lower than in the whole tissue. On the other hand, the lactate:pyruvate ratio, already very dissimilar in the two different cerebral preparations from normoxic dogs (about 19.1 in frozen cortical tissues and about 3.8 in incubated synaptosomal pellets), was increased by hypoxia with different magnifications in the two quoted preparations: ×4.0 in frozen cortical tissues and × 1.2 in incubated synaptosomal pellets.

As concerns the energy mediators, in the frozen cerebral cortex hypoxia induced a de-

Table I. Motor area of cerebral cortex from normocapnic beagle dogs in hypovolemic hypotension (MABP = 55 ± 4 mm Hg)

Metabolite or ratio	Frozen cortical tissues		Synaptosomal pellets	
	normoxia	hypoxia	normoxia	hypoxia
ATP	2.38 ± 0.04	1.79 ± 0.12*	5.45 ± 0.10	5.06 ± 0.20
ADP	0.41 ± 0.02	0.59 ± 0.02*	1.74 ± 0.05	1.82 ± 0.10
AMP	0.07 ± 0.01	0.53 ± 0.10*	0.43 ± 0.02	0.56 ± 0.02*
Σ Adenine nucleotides	2.86 ± 0.01	2.91 ± 0.03	7.62 ± 0.07	7.44 ± 0.12
Energy charge	0.903 ± 0.003	0.715 ± 0.032*	0.829 ± 0.003	0.801 ± 0.009*
Creatine phosphate	4.62 ± 0.11	2.11 ± 0.16*	5.42 ± 0.10	4.20 ± 0.28*
Pyruvate	0.111 ± 0.004	0.269 ± 0.024*	5.82 ± 0.15	7.03 ± 0.21*
Lactate	2.13 ± 0.16	20.59 ± 1.36*	22.08 ± 0.56	33.06 ± 1.04*
Lactate:pyruvate	19.09 ± 1.12	77.06 ± 3.05*	3.83 ± 0.12	4.76 ± 0.20*

Results are expressed as mean values ± SE.

Metabolite contents evaluated: (a) in frozen cortical tissues (μmol/g); (b) in synaptosomal pellets after further incubation for 10 min at 24 °C (nmol/mg protein). Behavior in normoxia and after 15 min of hypoxemia (PaO_2 = 17–19 mm Hg).

* Differs from normoxic animals ($p < 0.05$): Student's t test.

Table II. Motor area of cerebral cortex from normocapnic beagle dogs in hypovolemic hypotension (MABP = 55 ± 4 mm Hg)

Metabolite or ratio	Normoxic untreated animals (20)	Normoxic animals treated with intracarotid perfusion (0.1 ml · min^{-1} · kg^{-1} for 30 min) with		
		phenobarbital 5×10^{-3} *M* (7)	papaverine 1×10^{-4} *M* (7)	(–)eburnamonine 5×10^{-4} *M* (6)
ATP	5.45 ± 0.10	14.05 ± 0.92*	4.91 ± 0.35	5.26 ± 0.21
ADP	1.74 ± 0.05	2.24 ± 0.21*	1.62 ± 0.12	1.91 ± 0.16
AMP	0.43 ± 0.02	0.23 ± 0.03*	0.48 ± 0.03	0.40 ± 0.05
Σ Adenine nucleotides	7.62 ± 0.07	16.53 ± 0.75*	7.03 ± 0.23	7.57 ± 0.08
Energy charge	0.829 ± 0.003	0.916 ± 0.009*	0.811 ± 0.012	0.820 ± 0.011
Creatine phosphate	5.42 ± 0.10	13.02 ± 0.94*	5.10 ± 0.37	5.58 ± 0.30
Pyruvate	5.82 ± 0.15	2.92 ± 0.45*	6.08 ± 0.45	5.97 ± 0.61
Lactate	22.08 ± 0.56	18.24 ± 1.23	24.76 ± 1.96	25.80 ± 2.19
Lactate:pyruvate	3.83 ± 0.12	7.20 ± 1.08*	4.06 ± 0.14	4.41 ± 0.35

Results are expressed as mean values ± SE for the number of experiments indicated in parentheses.

Metabolite contents (nmol/mg protein) in synaptosomal pellets (after incubation for 10 min at 24 °C) obtained from untreated and treated normoxic animals.

* Differs from normoxic untreated animals ($p < 0.05$): Dunnett's test.

crease of ATP (× 0.75) and an increase of both ADP (× 1.4) and AMP (× 7.6), the energy charge potential being appreciably decreased (× 0.8). On the contrary, in incubated synaptosomal pellets hypoxia did not induce changes on ATP and ADP contents, only AMP being increased (× 1.3) even if to a much lower extent than on the whole cerebral tissue. In the incubated synaptosomal pellets the energy charge potential was already lower than in the whole cerebral cortex from normoxic beagle dogs, and also showed a lower decrease by hypoxia (× 0.97). In the same way, creatine phosphate decrease by hypoxia was much higher (× 0.46) in the whole cerebral cortex than in the incubated synaptosomal pellets (× 0.77).

Effects on Synaptosomes of the Pharmacological Treatment in Normocapnic Normoxic Animals

Table II summarizes the content of various metabolites and energy mediators in synaptosomes isolated from the motor area of the cerebral cortex of untreated and treated normoxic beagle dogs. In respect to the untreated animals, the contents of ATP and creatine phosphate were much higher in the synaptosomal pellets from the cerebral cortex of phenobarbital-treated dogs, while the content of AMP was lower, ADP being only slightly higher. Consequently both the total adenine nucleotide content and the energy charge potential were higher in the synaptosomal preparations from phenobarbital-perfused dogs, in comparison with those from untreated animals. The contents of lactate and, particularly, of pyruvate were lower in synaptosomes from phenobarbital-treated animals: this behavior lead to an increase in the lactate:pyruvate ratio. The perfusion with papaverine or (–)eburnamonine did not induce any significant change in the metabolite content of the incubated synaptosomal preparations.

Effects on Synaptosomes of the Pharmacological Treatment in Normocapnic Hypoxic Animals

It can be seen in table III that, in respect to the hypoxic untreated dogs, in synaptosomes from the cerebral cortex of hypoxic phenobarbital- and (–)eburnamonine-treated dogs, the contents of ATP and creatine phosphate were higher, while the content of AMP was lower, ADP being unchanged. Consequently, both the total adenine nucleotide contents and the energy charge potentials were higher in the synaptosomal preparations from hypoxic phenobarbital- and (–)eburnamonine-perfused dogs in comparison with those from hypoxic untreated animals, papaverine perfusion being without any action. In addition the contents of ATP and creatine phosphate, the total adenine nucleotide contents, and the energy charge potentials were higher in the synaptosomal preparations from hypoxic phenobarbital- and (–)eburnamonine-perfused dogs than in preparations from normoxic animals (table III vs. table I).

The contents of lactate and pyruvate were lower in synaptosomal preparations from the motor area of the cerebral cortex of hypoxic phenobarbital-perfused dogs in respect to hypoxic untreated ones. In synaptosomes from (–)eburnamonine- and papaverine-treated animals, the contents of pyruvate and lactate, within experimental error, were the same as those from hypoxic untreated animals, with the exception of the pyruvate synaptosomal content in papaverine-perfused dogs which was slightly higher.

Table III. Motor area of cerebral cortex from normocapnic beagle dogs in hypovolemic hypotension (MABP = 55 ± 4 mm Hg)

Metabolite or ratio	Hypoxic untreated animals (16)	Hypoxic animals treated with intracarotid perfusion (0.1 ml · min^{-1} · kg^{-1} for 15 + 15 min) with		
		phenobarbital 5×10^{-3} *M* (6)	papaverine 1×10^{-4} *M* (5)	(–)eburnamonine 5×10^{-4} *M* (5)
ATP	5.06 ± 0.20	11.23 ± 0.46*	4.73 ± 0.21	7.98 ± 0.51*
ADP	1.82 ± 0.10	1.66 ± 0.15	1.97 ± 0.21	1.84 ± 0.20
AMP	0.56 ± 0.02	0.30 ± 0.03*	0.63 ± 0.06	0.38 ± 0.03*
Σ Adenine nucleotides	7.44 ± 0.12	13.20 ± 0.32*	7.33 ± 0.26	10.20 ± 0.56
Energy charge	0.801 ± 0.009	0.913 ± 0.008*	0.779 ± 0.005	0.872 ± 0.011
Creatine phosphate	4.20 ± 0.28	7.96 ± 0.34*	3.83 ± 0.25	6.02 ± 0.31*
Pyruvate	7.03 ± 0.21	2.65 ± 0.20*	8.21 ± 0.42*	6.63 ± 0.32
Lactate	33.06 ± 1.04	14.36 ± 0.70*	34.63 ± 1.69	34.81 ± 1.23
Lactate:pyruvate	4.76 ± 0.20	5.54 ± 0.44	4.26 ± 0.29	5.28 ± 0.24

Results are expressed as mean values ± SE for the number of experiments indicated in parentheses.

Metabolites content (nmol/mg protein) in synaptosomal pellets (after incubation for 10 min at 24 °C) obtained from untreated or pretreated (for 15 min) and treated hypoxic animals (PaO_2 = 17–19 mm Hg, for 15 min).

* Differs from hypoxic untreated animals ($p < 0.05$): Dunnett's test.

Table IV. Oxygen consumption rates and cytochromes levels in synaptosomal pellets from the motor area of the cerebral cortex of normoxic and hypoxic beagle dogs in hypovolemic hypotension (MABP = 55 ± 4 mm Hg)

Biochemical parameters	Normoxic animals (10)	Hypoxic animals treated with intracarotid perfusion (0.1 ml · min^{-1} · kg^{-1} for 15 + 15 min) with			
		saline solution (10)	phenobarbital 5×10^{-3} *M* (6)	papaverine 1×10^{-4} *M* (5)	(–)eburnamonine 5×10^{-4} *M* (5)
Oxygen consumption rate nmol/min/mg protein	2.91 ± 0.23*	1.65 ± 0.36	1.78 ± 0.25	1.57 ± 0.36	1.73 ± 0.29
Cytochrome c nmol/mg protein	0.13 ± 0.02*	0.09 ± 0.02	0.04 ± 0.01*	0.10 ± 0.03	0.06 ± 0.01*
Cytochrome a nmol/mg protein	0.10 ± 0.01*	0.07 ± 0.01	0.03 ± 0.00*	0.08 ± 0.01	0.04 ± 0.00*

Results are expressed as mean values ± SE for the number of experiments indicated in parentheses.

* Differs from hypoxic untreated animals ($p < 0.05$): Dunnett's test.

Discussion

The present research was aimed at depicting how the brain synapses are sensitive to hypoxia and if some pharmacological agents – such as phenobarbital, papaverine, (–)eburnamonine – might prevent or reverse the effects of hypoxic damage. The choice of synaptosomal pellets was justified because of: (1) their sensitivity to hypoxia; (2) the availability of synaptosomal preparations which were metabolically active. Preliminarily, the effects of hypoxia on the whole tissue from the motor area of cerebral cortex (of beagle dogs in hypovolemic hypotension: MABP = 55 ± 5 mm Hg) were compared with the effects induced on the same parameters evaluated in synaptosomal pellets from the controlateral area. In the former case, the approach identified the actual metabolic changes induced by hypoxia itself while, in the latter case, the approach identified what synaptosomes remainded from the hypoxic damage and that could not be reversed during the 10 min of incubation at 24 °C.

In normoxia, the results shown in table I indicate that, in respect to the controlateral whole tissue, synaptosomes exhibit: (1) lower lactate:pyruvate ratio; (2) lower energy charge potential; (3) different ATP:ADP:AMP ratios. Furthermore, after 15 min of hypoxemia (PaO_2 = 17–19 mm Hg), the results shown in table I indicate that, in respect to the controlateral whole tissue, synaptosomes exhibit: (1) much lower increase of lactate:pyruvate ratio; (2) a lower decrease of creatine phosphate content; (3) no changes in ATP and ADP content; (4) much lower increase in AMP content. The drug's action is discussed here only in correlation with the changes induced on the behavior of the incubated synaptosomal preparations from brain of normoxic or hypoxic beagle dogs.

As indicated in tables II and III, papaverine was always inactive, while (–)eburnamonine increased the synaptosomal phosphorylation state in hypoxic animals, being ineffective on the glycolytic metabolites tested. Phenobarbital increased the synaptosomal phosphorylation state both in normoxic and hypoxic animals, and was effective also on the glycolytic metabolites studied. Furthermore, it can be seen in table IV that although the oxygen uptake was the same in the synaptosomal preparations from the cerebral cortex of hypoxic untreated or phenobarbital- and (–)eburnamonine-treated dogs, the cytochrome c and a contents were lower in the latter preparations. This indicates that the turnover rates for cytochromes c and a were higher in synaptosomes from brains of phenobarbital- or (–)eburnamonine-treated dogs. This behavior is consistent with the increased phosphorylation state in the synaptosomal preparations from the motor area of cerebral cortex of phenobarbital- and (–)eburnamonine-treated dogs. As concerns the low values of cytochrome contents in the synaptosomes from phenobarbital- and (–)eburnamonine-treated animals, two possible explanations are: (1) drugs induced changes in the rate of synthesis and/or degradation of cytochromes, in spite of the time scale of minutes involved in the present research; (2) drugs induced changes in the releasing process which leads to the formation of synaptosomes, so that vesicles contained a different number of intrasynaptosomal mitochondria. However, drug treatment and/or ischemia induced on synaptosomes and on mitochondria different and complex effects on the mitochondrial marker enzymatic activities [*Villa* et al., in press]. In any case, the data reported here (table IV) show that synaptosomal preparations from hypoxic treated or untreated dogs exhibit lower rates of oxygen consumption than do synaptosomes from untreated normoxic animals.

On the other hand, both the energy charge potential and the creatine phosphate storage were found to be higher in the synaptosomes isolated from the cerebral cortex of dogs that had been treated with phenobarbital or (–)eburnamonine. The three most likely explanations for this finding are related to some specific properties of the two drugs, such as: (1) stabilization of synaptosomal plasma membrane; (2) lowering of the body or brain temperature; (3) inhibition of sympathetic discharge that occurs during the withdrawal of the cerebral samples. In any case, the evaluated contents of adenine nucleotides reflect their free, cytosolic concentration, the binding of nucleotides (eventually affecting ADP) or the compartmentation (eventually affecting both mitochondria and intrasynaptic vesicles) not contributing a large error to the evaluations [*Rafalowska* et al., 1980b].

References

Atkinson, D.E.: The energy charge of the adenylate pool as regulatory parameter. Interaction with feed-back modifiers. Biochemistry, N.Y. *7:* 4030–4034 (1968).

Benzi, G.: An analysis of the drugs acting on cerebral energy metabolism. Jap. J. Pharmac. *25:* 251–261 (1975).

Benzi, G.; Arrigoni, E.; Dagani, F.; Pastoris, O.; Villa, R.F.; Agnoli, A.: Cerebral energy state during or after hypoxia and complete or incomplete ischemia. J. appl. Physiol. *45:* 312–319 (1978).

Benzi, G.; Villa, R.F.: Adenyl cyclase system and cerebral energy state. J. Neurol. Neurosurg. Psychiat. *39:* 77–83 (1976).

Chance, B.; Cohen, P.; Jöbsis, F.; Schoener, B.: Intracellular oxidation-reduction states in vivo. Science *137:* 499–508 (1962).

Chance, B.; Schoener, B.: Correlation of oxidation-reduction changes of intracellular reduced pyridine nucleotide and changes in electroencephalogram of the rat in anoxia. Nature, Lond. *195:* 956–958 (1962).

Chance, B.; Schoener, B.; Schindler, F.: in Dickens, Neil, Oxygen in the animal organism, pp. 367–392 (Pergamon Press, Oxford 1964).

Czok, R.; Lamprecht, W.: Pyruvate, phosphoenolpyruvate and *D*-glycerate-2-phosphate; in Bergmeyer, Methods of enzymatic analysis, pp. 1446–1451 (Academic Press, New York 1974).

De Robertis, E.; Pellegrino de Iraldi, A.; Rodriguez de Lores Arnaiz, G.; Salganicoff, L.: Cholinergic and noncholinergic nerve endings in rat brain. J. Neurochem. *9:* 23–35 (1962).

Gray, E.G.; Whittaker, V.R.: The isolation of nerve endings from brain. An electron-microscopy study of cell fragments derived by homogenization and centrifugation. J. Anat. *26:* 79–87 (1962).

Grossman, R.G.; Williams, V.F.: Electrical activity and ultrastructure of cortical neurones and synapses in ischemia; in Brierley, Meldrum, Brain hypoxia, pp. 61–75 (Lippincott, Philadelphia 1971).

Gurdjian, E.S.; Stone, W.E.; Werbster, J.E.: Cerebral metabolism in hypoxia. Archs Neurol. Psychiat., Chicago *51:* 472–477 (1944).

Gutmann, I.; Wahlefeld, A.W.: *L*-Lactate. Determination with lactate dehydrogenase and NAD; in Bergmeyer, Methods of enzymatic analysis, pp. 1464–1468 (Academic Press, New York 1974).

Hindfelt, B.; Siesjö, B.K.: Cerebral effects of acute ammonia intoxication. I. The influence on intracellular and extracellular acid-base parameters. Scand. J. clin. Lab. Invest. *28:* 353–364 (1971).

Kogure, K.; Scheinberg, P.; Reinmuth, O.M., Fujishima, M.; Busto, R.: Mechanisms of cerebral vasodilatation in hypoxia. J. appl. Physiol. *29:* 223–229 (1970).

Jansson, S.-E.; Härkönen, M.H.; Helve, H.: Metabolic properties of nerve endings isolated from rat brain. Acta physiol. scand. *107:* 205–212 (1979).

Jaworek, D.; Gruber, W.; Bergmeyer, H.U.: Adenosine-5′-diphosphate and adenosine-5′-monophosphate; in Bergmeyer, Methods of enzymatic analysis, pp. 2127–2131 (Academic Press, New York 1974).

Lamprecht, W.; Stein, P.; Heinz, F.; Weisser, H.: Creatine phosphate. Determination with creatine kinase, hexokinase, and glucose-6-phosphate dehydrogenase; in Bergmeyer, Methods of enzymatic analysis, pp. 1777–1781 (Academic Press, New York 1974).

Lamprecht, W.; Trautschold, I.: Adenosine-5′-triphosphate. Determination with hexokinase and glucose-6-phosphate dehydrogenase; in Bergmeyer, Methods of enzymatic analysis, pp. 2101–2110 (Academic Press, New York 1974).

MacMillan, V.; Siesjö, B.K.: Critical oxygen tensions in the brain. Acta physiol. scand. *82:* 412–414 (1971).

Rafalowska, U.; Erecinska, M.; Wilson, D.F.: The effect of acute hypoxia on synaptosomes from rat brain. J. Neurochem. *34:* 1160–1167 (1980a).

Rafalowska, U.; Erecinska, M.; Wilson, D.F.: Energy metabolism in rat brain synaptosomes from nembutal-anesthetized and nonanesthetized animals. J. Neurochem. *34:* 1380–1386 (1980b).

Siesjö, B.K.; Nilsson, L.: The influence of arterial hypoxemia upon labile phosphates and upon extracellular and intracellular lactate and pyruvate concentrations in the rat brain. Scand. J. clin. Lab. Invest. *27:* 83–96 (1971).

Siesjö, B.K.; Plum, F.: Pathophysiology of anoxic brain damage; in Gaull, Biology of brain dysfunction, vol. 1, pp. 319–372 (1973).

Silver, I.A.: Local PO_2 in relation to intracellular pH, cell membrane potential and potassium leakage in hypoxia and shock. Adv. exp. Med. Biol. *37A:* 223–231 (1973).

Villa, R.F.; Benzi, G.; Curti, D.: The effect of ischemia and pharmacological treatment evaluated on synaptosomes and purified mitochondria from rat brain (in press).

G. Benzi, MD, Department of Science, Institute of Pharmacology, University of Pavia,
Piazza Botta, 11, I–27100 Pavia (Italy)

Eur. Neurol. *20:* 245–252 (1981)

Brain Enzymes and Ischemia

R.F. Villa

Department of Science, Institute of Pharmacology, University of Pavia, Italy

Key Words. Brain · Ischemia · Mitochondria · Synaptosomes · Enzymatic activities · Energy metabolism

Abstract. Changes in the maximal rate of some cerebral enzymatic activities related to 400ene transduction and neurotransmission (lactate dehydrogenase; citrate synthase and malate dehydrogenase; total NADH-cytochrome c reductase and cytochrome oxidase; glutamate dehydrogenase; acetylcholine esterase) were assayed both in the crude or purified mitochondrial fraction and in the crude synaptosomal fraction from rat whole brain or cerebral cortex. The evaluations were performed in rats before and after a postdecapitative normothermic ischemia of 5, 10, 20 and 40 min duration. Modifications observed in some of these activities were discussed for comparison with other experimental results from different researchers. At present no definite conclusions can be drawn, but certainly the observed modifications in activity of enzymes are not passive but expression of deranged metabolism of ischemic neurons.

Introduction

During these last few years, it has been pointed out that biochemical techniques can be conveniently used in pharmacological and physiopathological investigations aimed at elucidating the mechanisms of action of drugs and interactions between physiopathological events and biochemical modifications [1–5].

As regards the effects of complete ischemia in the rat, they include changes in some amino acids acting as transmitters in the central nervous system and changes in substrates, intermediates and end products of glycolysis, Krebs' cycle, nerve transmission and amino acid metabolism. Nevertheless, the neurochemical factors accounting for the ischemic vulnerability of the brain are not completely understood – for a review, see *Siesjö* [6].

Whether the cerebral blood flow is stopped (e.g. vascular occlusion, increased intracranial pressure, asystole or severe arterial hypotension) or cut off (e.g., decapitation), the brain becomes a closed thermodynamic system in which the energy transduction is limited to the degradation of endogenous substrates. The concept of irreversible damage occurring in normothermic animals after a period of complete ischemia for more than 5–10 min has been previously postulated for a review, see *Mrsulja* et al. [7]. Nevertheless, more recent experimental data show that, under particular conditions, the neuronal activity may be reestablished after longer ischemic periods [8, 9].

In any case, in regard to the energy transduction, data concerning the behavior of enzymatic activities of brain during ischemia [7, 10–13] are disordered and recorded at different periods of ischemic damage. Therefore

Table I. Enzymatic activities (μmol · min^{-1} · mg $protein^{-1}$) related to energy transduction evaluated on homogenate in toto and crude mitochondrial fractions from the whole brain of control and ischemic rats (mean ± SEM)

Fraction	Conditions		
	saline solution	ischemia 5 min	saline solution
Homogenate			
Lactate dehydrogenase	0.786 ± 0.018 (9)	0.774 ± 0.016 (9)	0.827 ± 0.019 (7)
Malate dehydrogenase	1.681 ± 0.030 (9)	1.623 ± 0.048 (9)	1.725 ± 0.035 (9)
NADH-cytochrome reductase	0.046 ± 0.002 (8)	0.044 ± 0.001 (8)	0.050 ± 0.001 (8)
Cytochrome oxidase	0.223 ± 0.009 (7)	0.301 ± 0.015** (16)	0.220 ± 0.007 (8)
Acetylcholine esterase	0.116 ± 0.002 (10)	0.116 ± 0.003 (10)	0.114 ± 0.002 (9)
Crude mitochondria			
Citrate synthase	0.097 ± 0.004 (11)	0.096 ± 0.004 (11)	0.098 ± 0.006 (7)
Malate dehydrogenase	1.771 ± 0.042 (10)	1.679 ± 0.047 (10)	1.836 ± 0.021 (9)
NADH-cytochrome reductase	0.144 ± 0.002 (9)	0.123 ± 0.003*** (19)	0.153 ± 0.004 (7)
Cytochrome oxidase	1.238 ± 0.020 (11)	1.121 ± 0.032 (18)	1.208 ± 0.034 (8)
Glutamate dehydrogenase	0.130 ± 0.023 (8)	0.133 ± 0.003 (8)	0.131 ± 0.024 (6)

Number of animals for each group in brackets.
Differs from control rats: * $p < 0.05$; ** $p < 0.02$; *** $p < 0.01$ (Student's t test).

this work is intended to overcome it, besides being aimed at detecting changes in the maximal rate of some enzymatic activities: (a) at short and regular intervals of time (after 5, 10, 20 and 40 min of postdecapitative ischemia); (b) in representative subcellular fractions (homogenate, crude or purified mitochondria and crude synaptosomes); (c) evaluating enzyme activities representative of the glycolytic pathway (lactate dehydrogenase), Krebs' cycle (citrate synthase, malate dehydrogenase), electron transport chain (total NADH-cytochrome c reductase, cytochrome oxidase), amino acid metabolism (glutamate dehydrogenase) and neurotransmission (acetylcholine esterase).

ischemia 10 min	saline solution	ischemia 20 min	saline solution	ischemia 40 min
0.794 ± 0.020 (7)	0.772 ± 0.021 (9)	0.751 ± 0.029 (9)	0.791 ± 0.014 (12)	0.760 ± 0.016 (12)
1.640 ± 0.057 (9)	1.651 ± 0.042 (9)	1.527 ± 0.033* (9)	1.723 ± 0.031 (13)	1.665 ± 0.034 (12)
0.048 ± 0.002 (8)	0.048 ± 0.002 (8)	0.049 ± 0.003 (8)	0.047 ± 0.001 (11)	0.048 ± 0.002 (11)
0.295 ± 0.019*** (8)	0.211 ± 0.007 (9)	0.376 ± 0.014*** (14)	0.204 ± 0.007 (6)	0.335 ± 0.020*** (10)
0.106 ± 0.003* (9)	0.118 ± 0.003 (8)	0.116 ± 0.003 (8)	0.114 ± 0.002 (11)	0.114 ± 0.003 (12)
0.120 ± 0.006** (9)	0.096 ± 0.004 (11)	0.128 ± 0.008*** (11)	0.097 ± 0.009 (12)	0.134 ± 0.009*** (12)
1.813 ± 0.039 (9)	1.726 ± 0.041 (9)	1.752 ± 0.044 (11)	1.782 ± 0.030 (13)	1.789 ± 0.051 (13)
0.142 ± 0.008 (7)	0.132 ± 0.006 (11)	0.155 ± 0.010 (11)	0.127 ± 0.009 (6)	0.153 ± 0.012 (10)
1.285 ± 0.042 (8)	1.168 ± 0.023 (14)	1.247 ± 0.041 (18)	1.327 ± 0.039 (9)	1.023 ± 0.038* (12)
0.152 ± 0.011 (6)	0.178 ± 0.011 (9)	0.222 ± 0.012** (12)	0.136 ± 0.006 (11)	0.146 ± 0.007 (11)

Materials and Methods

The experiments were performed on female Sprague Dawley rats, weighing 250 ± 10 g, fasted overnight before use. The animals were selected according to randomized experimental procedures, kept from birth under standard cycling and caging conditions (temperature: 22 ± 1 °C; relative humidity: 60 ± 3%; lighting cycle: 12 h light and 12 h darkness; low noise disturbances), fed a standard pellet diet and water ad libitum, housed 3 and subsequently 2 per cage. The time course of ischemia performed in the lots was established by permutation tables.

Postdecapitative normothermic ischemia [10] was performed for 5, 10, 20 and 40 min, always starting at 10:00 a.m., because of circadian changes in cerebral enzymatic activities. At the set time, the brain was removed from the skull within 15 s and immersed in a cold 0.32 *M* sucrose solution. All manipulations were performed in a precooled box at 0–5 °C. The cerebral cortex was isolated, then immersed in a cold 0.32 *M* sucrose solution and homogenized (Potter-Braun S homogenizer), with a Teflon pestle rotating at 1,000 r.p.m. (electronic control) for 30 s, with two strokes up and down. In the experiments with whole brain, the brain was submitted to the same procedure. The homogenate of whole brain and/or cerebral cortex was submitted to differential centrifugation [14] for isolating the crude and/or purified mitochondrial fraction and the crude synaptosomal fraction. Three centrifugations at 900 *g* were performed to remove nuclei. The crude mitochondrial fraction was obtained by two centrifugations at 11,500 *g* for 30 min (Beckman J-21C Supercentrifuge, rotor J20). The crude mitochondrial fraction was subsequently layered on discontinuous sucrose gradient (experiments with cerebral cortex) and centrifuged for 2 h at 50,000 *g* (Beckman L5-50 Ultracentrifuge, rotor SW 50.1) for the isolation of the purified mitochondrial fraction and crude synaptosomal fraction [14]. The synaptosomal fraction was removed by aspiration and then pelletted at 50,000 *g* for 30 min. All fractions were suspended in a 0.32 *M* sucrose solution and proteins were dosed [15]. The maximal rate of the following enzymatic activities were evaluated on samples of crude and/or purified mitochondrial fraction: citrate synthase (citrate oxaloacetate-lyase, EC 4.1.3.7) [16]; malate dehydrogenase (*L*-malate: NAD^+ oxidoreductase, EC 1.1.1.37) [17]; total NADH-cytochrome c reductase (NADH cytochrome c: oxygen oxidoreductase, EC 1.6.99.3) [18]; cytochrome oxidase (ferrocytochrome c: oxygen oxidoreductase, EC 1.9.3.1) [19, 20]; glutamate dehydrogenase (*L*-glutamate: NAD^+ oxidoreductase, deaminating, EC 1.4.1.3) [16]. On crude synaptosomal fraction samples from the brain cortex, the maximal rate of malate dehydrogenase [17], lactate dehydrogenase (*L*-lactate: NAD^+ oxidoreductase, EC 1.1.1.27) [21] and acetylcholinesterase (acetylcholine hydrolase, EC 3.1.1.7) [22] were also evaluated; on whole brain homogenate, lactate dehydrogenase and acetylcholinesterase were also assayed. Enzymatic activities were measured by graphic recordings for at least 3 min (Beckman 25 Recording Spectrophotometer) and expressed as specific activities. Each value was calculated from two determinations performed blindly on the same sample. Because of seasonal variations in the enzymatic activities, the groups of ischemic rats, treated with saline or submitted to experimental physiopathological conditions, were compared with their own group of controls at each individual time of ischemia. For statistical analysis, Student's t test was applied.

Results

Table I shows the results concerning the enzymatic activities evaluated in the brain homogenate as a whole and in the crude mitochondrial fraction from it, both under control conditions and after 5, 10, 20 and 40 min of total normothermic ischemia. The most significant event is the increased activity of cytochrome oxidase at all times during ischemia for homogenate, and in the mitochondrial fraction: first the increase of the activity of citrate synthase starting from 10 min of ischemia, and second the increase in the activity of glutamate dehydrogenase at 20 min. Slight and temporary falls in the activity of NADH-cytochrome c reductase at 5 min and of cytochrome oxidase at 40 min was also observed. The enzymatic activities evaluated on the purified mitochondrial fraction or the crude synaptosomal fraction from cerebral cortex are shown in table II. After 5 min of brain ischemia, the cerebral cortex showed a decrease both of total NADH-cytochrome c reductase activity in mitochondria and of acetylcholinesterase activity in synaptosomes. After 10 min, the cerebral cortex showed a decrease in malate dehydrogenase, NADH-cytochrome c reductase and glutamate dehydrogenase activities in the purified mitochondrial fraction. After 20 min, the cerebral cortex showed a decrease in malate dehydrogenase and total NADH-cytochrome reductase activities in mitochondria and a decrease of acetylcholinesterase activity in synaptosomes. Also after 40 min of brain ischemia, decreases of NADH-cytochrome c reductase activity in mitochondria and of acethylcholine esterase activity in synaptosomes were observed.

Discussion

The presented data relative to the behavior of enzymatic activities after various times of ischemia raise these questions: (a) do the observed changes in enzyme activities represent the passive outcome of membrane structures damage [3] or (b), on the contrary, are there active responses to the ischemic condition? As for the ischemic changes in the enzyme activities evaluated in the homogenate in toto of whole brain, the modification undergone by cytochrome oxidase can be ascribed to a modified redox state of cytoplasm, in agreement with previous findings of *Gromek and Pastuszko* [10] who, in evaluating the effect of changes of mitochondrial NADP-dependent isocitrate dehydrogenase during ischemia, suggested the existence of an unknown mechanism regulating the activity of enzymes at the level of the subcellular fraction in relation to the altered state of neurons. As concerns the mitochondrial fraction, among the enzymes related to Krebs' cycle, malate dehydrogenase decreased in activity only when activity was assayed at 10 and 20 min of ischemia in purified mitochondria, while citrate synthase increased its activity only when evaluated on crude mitochondria from whole brain. As concerns enzymes related to the electron transport chain, total NADH-cytochrome c reductase is the most sensitive to ischemia (decrease in activity from 0 to 40 min in purified and 5 min in crude mitochondria). Glutamate dehydrogenase exhibited a decrease in activity at time 10 min and/or 20 min of ischemia depending on the fraction assayed. At the synaptosomal level, only acetylcholinesterase decreased in activity from 0 to 40 min of ischemia, except at 10 min; however, at this time, enzyme activity decreased on homogenate. On the whole, these findings are consistent with the rearrangements of some enzymatic activities observed by other authors during cerebral ischemia. For example, the active form of pyruvate dehydrogenase was described to increase by about 40% after 3 min of ischemia [23], thus indicating an increase of about 90% of the total enzyme activity in ischemia. These events might explain the increase observed in this research of the activity of citrate synthase (whole brain). On the other hand, after 5 min of ischemia, changes in glucose-6-phosphatase distribution with a decrease in phosphatidylcholine and phosphatidylethanolamine content were found [13], indicating an activation of endogenous membrane-bound phospholipases in ischemia. Furthermore, 0.5–5 min of ischemia [24] resulted in a strong decrease of phospholipid content of guinea pig cerebral mitochondria, with an increase of both the free fatty acid pool and the level of malonyldialdehyde, indicating lipid peroxidation. In the present research, the ischemia (same model of the above-mentioned papers) resulted in a decrease in the activity of mitochondrial malate dehydrogenase and NADH-cytochrome c reductase and of acetylcholinesterase, involving the enzymes related to both the phosphorylation mechanism and neurotransmission.

Using another model of complete ischemia (increase in CSF pressure; 30 min) it was demonstrated [25] that, after recirculation, brain mitochondria showed extensive functional recovery with normalization of respiratory control ratio as well as of state 3 and maximal phosphorylation rates.

Therefore, the analysis of the present results and of the literature data allows one to suggest the existence in the brain of a variety of interrelated and intriguing factors implicated in the ischemia-induced changes in the maximal rate of mitochondrial enzymatic activities connected with energy transduction as well as with other integrated functions of neurons. In any case, these results are far

Table II. Enzymatic activities (μmol · min^{-1} · mg $protein^{-1}$) related to energy transduction evaluated on purified mitochondrial fractions from the cerebral cortex of control and ischemic rats (mean ± SEM)

Fraction	Conditions		
	saline solution	ischemia 5 min	saline solution
Purified mitochondria			
Citrate synthase	0.233 ± 0.010 (15)	0.230 ± 0.008 (15)	0.299 ± 0.015 (9)
Malate dehydrogenase	3.097 ± 0.060 (15)	3.058 ± 0.055 (15)	2.931 ± 0.084 (9)
NADH-cytochrome reductase	0.305 ± 0.011 (19)	0.256 ± 0.008*** (18)	0.274 ± 0.017 (7)
Cytochrome oxidase	2.072 ± 0.066 (14)	1.917 ± 0.051 (14)	1.834 ± 0.137 (7)
Glutamate dehydrogenase	0.276 ± 0.006 (13)	0.279 ± 0.008 (13)	0.349 ± 0.016 (8)
Crude synaptosomes			
Lactate dehydrogenase	0.644 ± 0.028 (16)	0.590 ± 0.027 (16)	0.630 ± 0.037 (9)
Malate dehydrogenase	1.734 ± 0.113 (13)	1.635 ± 0.108 (15)	1.578 ± 0.088 (9)
Acetylcholine esterase	0.137 ± 0.004 (17)	0.110 ± 0.005*** (17)	0.153 ± 0.007 (11)

Number of animals for each group in brackets.
Differs from control rats: * $p < 0.05$; ** $p < 0.02$; *** $p < 0.01$ (Student's t test).

from conclusive and research is in progress to study the effect of ischemia on brain enzymes related to energy transduction on several subfractions from various areas of the rat brain. In fact, the fractionation may be used to discriminate the changes recorded on enzyme activities, in many cases due to the complex rearrangement of these enzymes in subcellular compartments. In addition, the use of pharmacological agents may be useful for the explanation of changes observed in cerebral enzymes during ischemia.

References

1 Benzi, G.; Villa, R.F.: Adenyl cyclase system and cerebral energy state. J. Neurol. Neurosurg. Psychiat. *39:* 77–83 (1976).

2 Villa, R.F.; Strada, P.; Barbieri, G.: A comparative study on some mitochondrial enzymes from rat brain. Farmaco *32:* 192–196 (1977).

3 Villa, R.F.; Strada, P.; Dagani, F.; Benzi, G.: Magnification of some enzymatic activities of brain cortex subfractions. Biochem. Pharmac. *27:* 2278–2280 (1978).

4 Villa, R.F.; Strada, P.; Marzatico, F.; Dagani, F.: Effect of (–)eburnamonine, papaverine and UDP-

ischemia 10 min	saline solution	ischemia 20 min	saline solution	ischemia 40 min
0.186 ± 0.013 (11)	0.221 ± 0.008 (10)	0.193 ± 0.018 (6)	0.275 ± 0.020 (8)	0.240 ± 0.027 (6)
2.509 ± 0.055*** (12)	3.036 ± 0.069 (9)	2.495 ± 0.127*** (6)	2.904 ± 0.088 (9)	2.784 ± 0.084 (6)
0.195 ± 0.013*** (7)	0.258 ± 0.005 (9)	0.155 ± 0.009*** (7)	0.351 ± 0.025 (9)	0.226 ± 0.024*** (7)
1.488 ± 0.156 (8)	1.645 ± 0.044 (10)	1.550 ± 0.149 (7)	1.844 ± 0.140 (7)	1.558 ± 0.102 (7)
0.292 ± 0.014* (13)	0.325 ± 0.015 (10)	0.296 ± 0.025 (7)	0.395 ± 0.027 (8)	0.331 ± 0.018 (7)
0.570 ± 0.028 (10)	0.527 ± 0.029 (10)	0.608 ± 0.061 (6)	0.525 ± 0.024 (8)	0.543 ± 0.032 (7)
1.400 ± 0.086 (11)	1.429 ± 0.075 (8)	1.298 ± 0.102 (7)	1.473 ± 0.079 (6)	1.347 ± 0.092 (7)
0.132 ± 0.007 (11)	0.137 ± 0.005 (11)	0.111 ± 0.010* (8)	0.122 ± 0.001 (9)	0.087 ± 0.001** (8)

glucose on cerebral energy state during and after experimental hypoxia and ischemia in beagle dog. Eur. Neurol. *17:* 97–112 (1978).
5 Benzi, G.; Arrigoni, E.; Dagani, F.; Marzatico, F.; Curti, D.; Manzini, A.; Villa, R.F.: Effect of chronic treatment with some drugs on enzymatic activities of the rat brain. Biochem. Pharmac. *28:* 2703–2708 (1979).
6 Siesjö, B.K.: Brain energy metabolism (Wiley, New York 1978).
7 Mrsulja, B.B.; Rakic, L.J.M.; Klatzo, I.; Spatz, M.: Pathophysiology of cerebral energy metabolism (Plenum Press, New York 1979).
8 Ljunggren, B.; Ratcheson, R.A.; Siesjö, B.K.: Cerebral metabolic state following compression ischemia. Brain Res. *73:* 291–307 (1974).
9 Nordström, C.H.; Rehncrona, S.; Siesjö, B.K.: Restitution of cerebral energy state as well as of glycolytic metabolites, citric acid cycle intermediates and associated amino acids after 30 minutes of complete ischemia in rats anaesthetized with nitrous oxide or phenobarbital. J. Neurochem. *30:* 479–486 (1978).
10 Gromek, A.; Pastuszko, A.: The localization of mitochondrial NADP-dependent isocitrate dehydrogenase in normal and hypoxic conditions. J. Neurochem. *28:* 429–433 (1977).
11 Schwartz, J.P.; Mrsulja, B.B.; Mrsulja, B.J.; Passonneau, J.V.; Klatzo, I.: Alterations of cyclic nucleotide-related enzymes and ATPase during unilateral ischemia and recirculation in gerbil cerebral cortex. J. Neurochem. *27:* 101–107 (1976).
12 Rossowska, M.; Zalewska, T.: Effect of hypoxia and ischemia on the distribution of protein in brain cellular fractions. Neurochem. Res. *4:* 15–23 (1979).
13 Rossowska, M.; Dabrowiecki, Z.: Effect of hypoxia and ischemia on the activity of glucose-6-phosphatase in guinea-pig brain. J. Neurochem. *30:* 1203–1204 (1978).
14 De Robertis, E.; Pellegrino de Iraldi, A.; Rodriguez de Lores Arnaiz, G.; Salganicoff, L.: Cholinergic and non-cholinergic nerve endings in rat brain. I. J. Neurochem. *9:* 23–35 (1962).
15 Lowry, O.H.; Rosebrough, N.J.; Farr, A.R.; Randall, R.J.: Protein measurement with the Folin phenol reagent. J. biol. Chem. *193:* 265–275 (1951).
16 Sugden, P.H.; Newsholme, E.A.: Activities of citrate synthase NAD^+-linked and $NADP^+$-linked isocitrate dehydrogenase, glutamate dehydrogenase, aspartate aminotransferase and alanine aminotransferase in nervous tissues from vertebrates and invertebrates. Biochem. J. *150:* 105–111 (1975).
17 Ochoa, S.: Maltae dehydrogenase from pig heart; in Colowick, Kaplan, Methods in enzymology, vol. 1, pp. 735–739 (Academic Press, New York 1955).
18 Nason, A.; Vasington, F.D.: Lipid dependent DPNH-cytochrome c reductase from mammalian skeletal and heart muscle; in Colowick, Kaplan, Methods in enzymology, vol. 6, pp. 409–415 (Academic Press, New York 1963).
19 Smith, L.: Spectrophotometric assay of cytochrome c oxidase; in Glick, Methods of biochemical analysis, vol. 2, pp. 427–435 (Wiley, New York 1955).
20 Wharton, D.C.; Tzagoloff, A.: Cytochrome oxidase from beef heart mitochondria; in Estabrook, Pullman, Methods in enzymology, vol. 10, pp. 245–250 (Academic Press, New York 1967).
21 Bergmeyer, H.U.; Bernt, E.: Lactate dehydrogenase; in Bergmeyer, Methods of enzymatic analysis, vol. 2, pp. 574–579 (Academic Press, New York 1974).
22 Ellman, G.L.; Courtney, K.D.; Anders, V.; Featherstone, R.M.: A new and rapid colorimetric determination of acetylcholinesterase activity. Biochem. Pharmac. *7:* 88–95 (1961).
23 Ksiezak, H.: Effect of hypoxia, ischemia and barbiturate anesthesia on interconversion of pyruvate dehydrogenase in guinea-pig brain. FEBS Lett. *63:* 149–153 (1976).
24 Majewska, M.D.; Strosznajder, J.; Lazarewicz, J.: Effect of ischemic anoxia and barbiturate anesthesia on free radical oxidation of mitochondrial phospholipids. Brain Res. *158:* 423–434 (1978).
25 Rehncrona, S.; Mela, L.; Siesjö, B.K.: Recovery of brain mitochondrial function in the rat after complete and incomplete cerebral ischemia. Stroke *10:* 437–445 (1979).

R.F. Villa, Department of Science, Institute of Pharmacology, University of Pavia, Pavia (Italy)

Eur. Neurol. *20:* 253–257 (1981)

Experimental Approach of Activity and Mechanism(s) of Action of Drugs Used in Cerebral Metabolic Insufficiency

Application to *l*-Eburnamonine

P. Linee[a] *M.A. Hollands*[b], *P. Quiniou*[a], *M. Gueguen*[c], *J.B. Le Polles*[a]

[a]Centre Recherches des Laboratoires Sobio, St. Grégoire, France; [b]Beecham Pharmaceuticals Research Center, Gt. Burgh, UK; [c]Centre Régional Transfusion Sanguine, Rennes, France

Key Words. Cerebral metabolic insufficiency · Drugs · *l*-Eburnamonine · Experimental activity

Abstract. The authors described an experimental approach, specially using oral administration, of drugs used in cerebral metabolic insufficiencies and its application to *l*-eburnamonine (*l*-EB). Administered orally, *l*-EB: (1) significantly increased the cerebral consumption of [^{14}C]-deoxyglucose in normoxic mice; (2) decreased the fall in cerebral energy charge (ECP) of rats after an acute normobaric hypoxia, and (3) stimulated the glycolysis of red blood cells (RBC) in healthy volunteers (repeated administrations) as demonstrated by important increases in 2,3-DPG and ATP, i.e., in factors involved in the bioavailability of oxygen (oxygen transport activity and RBC deformability). The results therefore demonstrate oral activity of *l*-EB in animals and man. They are in agreement with previous data showing cerebral metabolic stimulant and antihypoxic effects following parenteral administration, in animals. They allow to propose that *l*-EB acts both at cerebral and extracerebral levels and constitute objective biochemical proof of the activity of *l*-EB in man. The study of new drugs may be done using the same experimental approach.

Introduction

The study of drugs potentially active in the treatment of cerebral metabolic insufficiencies is very difficult. In animals, most of the methods use parenteral (i.v. or i.p.) administrations of drugs when these drugs are principally administered orally in patients. In man, objective proof of the activity of such drugs is uncommon. In order to contribute to resolve these problems, we propose some methods and their application to a known drug: *l*-eburnamonine.

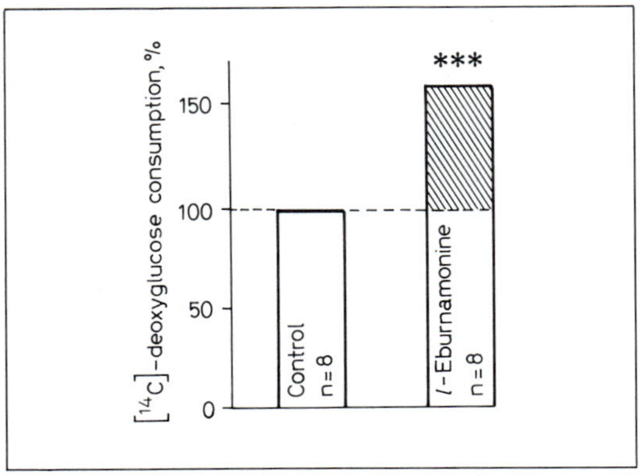

Fig. 1. Activity of *l*-eburnamonine (25 mg·kg^{-1}) administered orally 60 min before deoxyglucose on the [^{14}C]-deoxyglucose consumption by the whole brain of normoxic mice. *** $p < 0.001$.

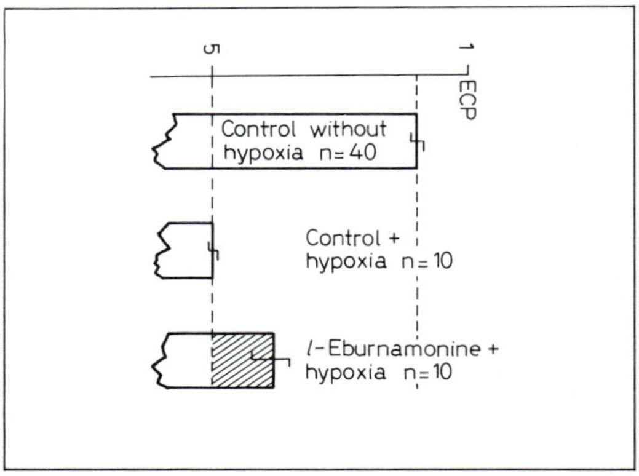

Fig. 2. Activity of *l*-eburnamonine (200 mg·kg^{-1}) administered orally on ECP in rats 30 min before an acute normobaric oxyprive hypoxia.

Experimental Methods

Cerebral [^{14}C]-Deoxyglucose Consumption in Normoxic Mice. The experimental procedure used was previously described [7]. *l*-Eburnamonine (25 mg·kg^{-1}) was administered orally 60 min before deoxyglucose (0.2 μCi intravenously). Mice were killed 30 min after deoxyglucose and the cerebral consumption was measured in the whole brain using a liquid scintillation method. Results were expressed in terms of changes (percent) in comparison with control mice.

Cerebral Energy Charge (ECP) in Rats after Acute Normobaric Hypoxia. According to *Atkinson* [1], ECP was measured in total frozen brain after killing rats by immersion in liquid nitrogen immediately after an acute normobaric hypoxia (pure gazeous nitrogen: 15 liters·min^{-1}during 90 s in a 5-liter desiccator). *l*-Eburnamonine (200 mg·kg^{-1}) was administered orally 30 min before hypoxia. ECP was measured in control rats without hypoxia, in control rats with hypoxia and in treated rats with hypoxia.

Red Blood Cells (RBC) 2,3-Diphosphoglycerate (2,3-DPG) and ATP in Human. 2,3-DPG (*Michal's* method [6], Boehringer Kit) and ATP (UV spectrophotometric method, Boehringer Kit) were measured in venous blood samples in 18 healthy volunteers (9 women, 9 men), before (d.0.), 1 and 4 days after drug administrations (d.1, d.4) and 2 days after stopping administrations (d.7). *l*-Eburnamonine (60 mg 3 times a day) was administered orally during 5 days.

Results

Cerebral [^{14}C]-Deoxyglucose Consumption. See figure 1. In normoxic mice, an oral administration of *l*-eburnamonine significantly increased the brain consumption of deoxyglucose.

ECP after Acute Hypoxia. See figure 2. Acute hypoxia induced a very important decrease of ECP in control rats; an oral administration of *l*-eburnamonine significantly reduced this decrease.

RBC 2,3-DPG and ATP. See figure 3. In healthy volunteers, *l*-eburnamonine (repeated oral administration) increased significantly the RBC 2,3-DPG and ATP levels.

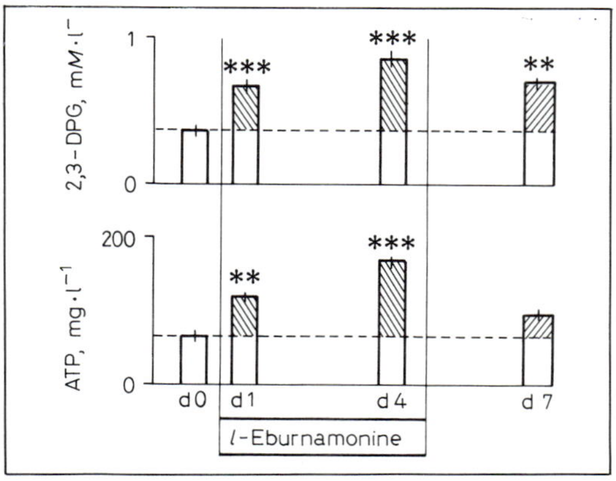

Fig. 3. Activity of *l*-eburnamonine (3 × 60 mg day/5 days) administered orally in 18 healthy volunteers on the RBC 2,3-DPG and ATP levels. *** $p < 0.001$; ** $p < 0.01$.

Such increases appeared as soon as the first day of treatment, were higher after 4 days and persisted 2 days after stopping drug administration.

Comments

These results with *l*-eburnamonine administered orally confirmed previously obtained data (see table I) demonstrating the cerebral oxygenating, cerebral metabolic stimulant and antihypoxic properties of this drug. *l*-Eburnamonine, administered by parenteral as well as by oral route, improves oxy-

Table I. Summary of the previous experimental data on *l*-eburnamonine

Test	Species	Route of administration	Results	References
CBF and cerebral metabolism	anesthetized dogs	i.v. perfusion	no changes in CBF, increase in O_2 and glucose supply, extraction and consumption	[3]
Cortical pO_2	rabbits	i.v.	increase	[4]
Antihypoxic				
KCN-induced histotoxic hypoxia	mice	orally	increase of survival time	personal work
Acute hypobaric hypoxia	mice	i.p.	increase of survival time	[5]
	rats	i.p.	memory retention (passive avoidance conditioning; 2 compartments box test)	[5]
Acute and reiterate asphyxia	curarized rats	i.v. perfusion	decrease of EEG disorders	[8]
Acute cerebral ischemia	curarized cats	i.v.	decrease of postischemic increase of thalamic-evoked potentials	[5]
Normobaric hypoxia + acute total cerebral ischemia	curarized dogs	i.a. perfusion	posthypoxic improvement of ECP recovery	[9]
Cerebral infarction	anesthetized cats	i.v. perfusion	decrease of cerebral infarction	[2]

Table II. Experimental 'profile' of 4 drugs

Activity	Drug			
	Dihydroergotoxine	*l*-Eburnamonine	Papaverine	Vincamine
CBF	↘↘	0	↗↗	↘
Cerebral metabolic stimulation	++	++	0	0
Antihypoxic	0	++	0	+

gen supply, oxygen cerebral extraction and consumption. The stimulation of the RBC glycolysis probably contributes to improving the oxygen availablility for nervous cells; as a matter of fact, 2,3-DPG is involved in the oxyhemoglobin dissociation processes and ATP is an important factor of the RBC deformability. On the other hand, the increases in RBC 2,3-DPG and ATP are objective biochemical proof of the oral activity of *l*-eburnamonine. *l*-Eburnamonine, administered by the parenteral as well by the oral route, also improves glucose cerebral extraction and consumption; it protects ECP. These activities explain the antihypoxic properties of this drug.

According to these results, it is possible to propose that *l*-eburnamonine acts both at the cerebral level as shown by effects on $CMRO_2$, CMR glucose, deoxyglucose consumption, ECP, and at the extracerebral level as shown by effect on RBC 2,3-DPG and ATP, increase in arterial pO_2 in dogs [3].

A same experimental approach may be used for new drugs. For example, table II summarizes some experimental 'profiles' obtained with the proposed methodology.

Of course, it is necessary to complete this experimental approach with more sophisticated methods, such as measurement of local cerebral metabolism using deoxyglucose autohistoradiography. On the other hand, it is important to know if an improvement of RBC parameters (2,3-DPG and ATP) is related to a decrease of the cerebral disturbances observed in the organic brain syndrome.

References

1 Atkinson, D.E.: Energy charge of adenylate pool as a regulatory factor. Interactions with feed back modifiers. Biochemistry *7:* 4030 (1968).

2 Fieschi, C.; Battistini, N.: Relazione sull preparato denominato CH–846 (vincamone). Personal commun. (1977).

3 Lacroix, P.; Quiniou, M.J.; Linee, P.; Le Polles, J.B.: Cerebral metabolic and hemodynamic properties of *l*-eburnamonine in the anesthetized dog. A comparison with vincamine. Arzneimittel-Forsch. *29:* 1094–1101 (1979).

4 Lacroix, P.; Plotkine, M.; Linee, P.; Le Polles, J.B.; Aurousseau, M.; Boulu, R.: Cerebral oxygenating properties of *l*-eburnamonine. 7th Int. Congr. Pharmacol.: Reims Satellite Symp. Cerebral Vascular Diseases (1978).

5 Linee, P.; Perrault, G.; Le Polles, J.B.; Lacroix, P.; Aurousseau, M.; Boulu, R.: Activité protectrice cérébrale de la *l*-éburnamonine étudiée sur 3 modèles d'aggression hypoxique aiguë. Comparaison avec la vincamine. Annls pharm. fr. *35:* 97–110 (1977).

6 Michal, G.: in Bergmeyer, Methods of enzymatic analysis, p. 1433 (Verlag Chemie, Weinheim/Academic Press, New York 1974).
7 Thomann, G.: Thèse Doct. Pharm. Paris (1977).
8 Van Den Driessche, J.; Linee, P.; Le Polles, J.B.; Lacroix, P.: Etude de la protection exercée par la *l*-éburnamonine vis-à-vis de l'anoxie asphyxique aiguë et itérative sur l'activité électrique cérébrale du rat curarisé. Comparaison avec la vincamine. C.r. Séanc. Soc. Biol. *171:* 1081–1088 (1977).
9 Villa, F.; Strada, P.; Marzatico, F.; Dagani, F.: Effects of (–)-eburnamonine, papaverine and UDP-glucose on cerebral energy state during and after experimental hypoxia in beagle dog. Eur. Neurol. *17:* suppl. 1, pp. 97–112 (1978).

P. Linee, PhD, Centre de Recherches
des Laboratoires Sobio, 4, rue du
Chesnay-Beauregard, F–35760 Saint-Grégoire
(France)

Eur. Neurol. *20:* 258–264 (1981)

Correlation of Local Blood Flow, Glucose Consumption and Probability of Necrosis following a Middle Cerebral Artery Occlusion in the Cat

I. Delage, D. Duverger, B. Gotti, E.T. MacKenzie

Department of Biology, LERS, Synthelabo, Bagneux, France

Key Words. Focal ischemia · Cerebral infarction · Neuropathological · Local cerebral blood flow · Cerebral glucose consumption

Abstract. At defined coronal sections, the surface area of infarcted tissue was measured 4 days after the occlusion of the middle cerebral artery in 11 cats. In groups of cats treated with ifenprodil (5.6 and 16.7 μg/kg · min over 3 h, 5 min after the occlusion), the infarcted surface was significantly decreased. The topographic localization of the infarction was studied in control and treated cats. This established necrosis was correlated with measures of focal cerebral blood flow and glucose consumption 3.5 h after the middle cerebral artery occlusion. Grey matter blood flow was universally low in untreated cats, but in cats treated with ifenprodil (5.6 μg/kg · min) cortical and caudate nucleus blood flow was 2–3 times greater, even in those regions that were later infarcted in the treated cats. Glucose consumption was similarly reduced in untreated cats but there was little difference between the control and drug-treated cats except in some areas where drug treatment appeared to further reduce the values for focal glucose consumption. These regions correlated with those in which infarction was later found in the cats treated with ifenprodil. It is hoped that such correlations between pathology, flow and metabolism could help in the search for effective pharmacotherapy of cerebrovascular disease.

Introduction

Occlusion of the middle cerebral artery in cats results in a reproducible infarction when studied 4 days later. The volume and distribution of this infarction can be significantly decreased by a number of drugs [*Bartholini* et al., 1980], one of which is ifenprodil. To further understand the mechanisms of this tissue sparing effect, focal cerebral blood flow and glucose consumption were measured, in control and ifenprodil-treated cats, 3.5 h after middle cerebral artery occlusion. These studies were correlated with the differences in pathology, noted 4 days after occlusion.

Methods and Results

A focal cerebral infarction was induced by the permanent occlusion of one middle cerebral artery in lightly anaesthetized cats. 4 days later, the brains were removed for histological analysis and the following parameters were assessed: surface area of necrotic tissue at defined coronal sections, the total volume of the infarction within a delineated brain region, and the topographic distribution of the ischemic tissue. The effects of ifenprodil on these parameters were studied by the intravenous infusion of the drug over 3 h; the infusion was first administered 5 min after middle cerebral artery occlusion. Three groups of cats were studied: 12 cats subjected to the saline alone; 13 cats treated with 5.6 μg/kg · min ifenprodil, and 13 cats treated with 16.7 μg/kg · min ifenprodil.

Pathology

Those cats treated with 5.6 and 16.7 μg/kg · min ifenprodil had a significantly lesser surface area and volume of brain tissue damaged by the middle cerebral artery occlusion when compared to their matched control group. The volume of irreversibly damaged brain was, on average, decreased by 24% ($p < 0.05$) in cats treated with 5.6 μg/kg · min ifenprodil; this amelioration was more evident in the caudal sections of cerebrum studied. In the cats treated with 16.7 μg/kg · min ifenprodil, the comparable decrease was 42% ($p < 0.001$).

In the ifenprodil-treated cats, the most clear and dose-related difference was the decreased distribution and incidence of cortical infarction when compared to untreated cats. In the rostral region studied, the probability of infarction in the corona radiata was apparently decreased considerably by ifenprodil treatment. However, there was no apparent difference in the vulnerability of the caudate nucleus to middle cerebral artery occlusion. Ifenprodil effected the greatest saving of cortical tissue in the more caudal of the sections studied (fig. 1), though white matter necrosis was still evident in the internal capsule.

Cerebral Blood Flow

Focal cerebral blood flow was measured in 4 untreated and 4 cats treated with ifenprodil (5.6 μg/kg · min). Blood flow was measured 3.5 h after the occlusion of the middle cerebral artery by the tissue uptake technique as modified for [^{14}C]-iodo-antipyrine. The tracer was infused over 30 s, after which saturated KCl was injected intravenously, the cat decapitated and the head frozen in liquid nitrogen. The brain was sectioned in a cryostat at –14 °C and, each 2 mm, samples taken at the sites indicated in figure 2.

Mean grey matter blood flow was markedly decreased in the untreated cats and, often, even the mean values were close to the critical ischemic threshold. In the caudate nucleus, the mean of all the measurements was 26 ± 6 ml/100 g · min in untreated cats as opposed to 73 ± 10 ml/100 g · min in ifenprodil-treated cats ($p < 0.01$). Over the convexity, mean grey matter blood flow was 19 ± 2 ml/100 g · min in untreated cats and 64 ± 3 ml/100 g · min in the treated group ($p < 0.001$). In the parasagittal region (where established necrosis is rare), blood flow was 37 ± 2 ml/100 g · min in the controls versus 72 ± 5 ml/100 g · min in treated cats ($p < 0.001$).

Glucose Consumption

Focal cerebral glucose consumption was measured, by the [^{14}C]-2-deoxyglucose technique, essentially as described by *Ginsberg* et

Coronal section

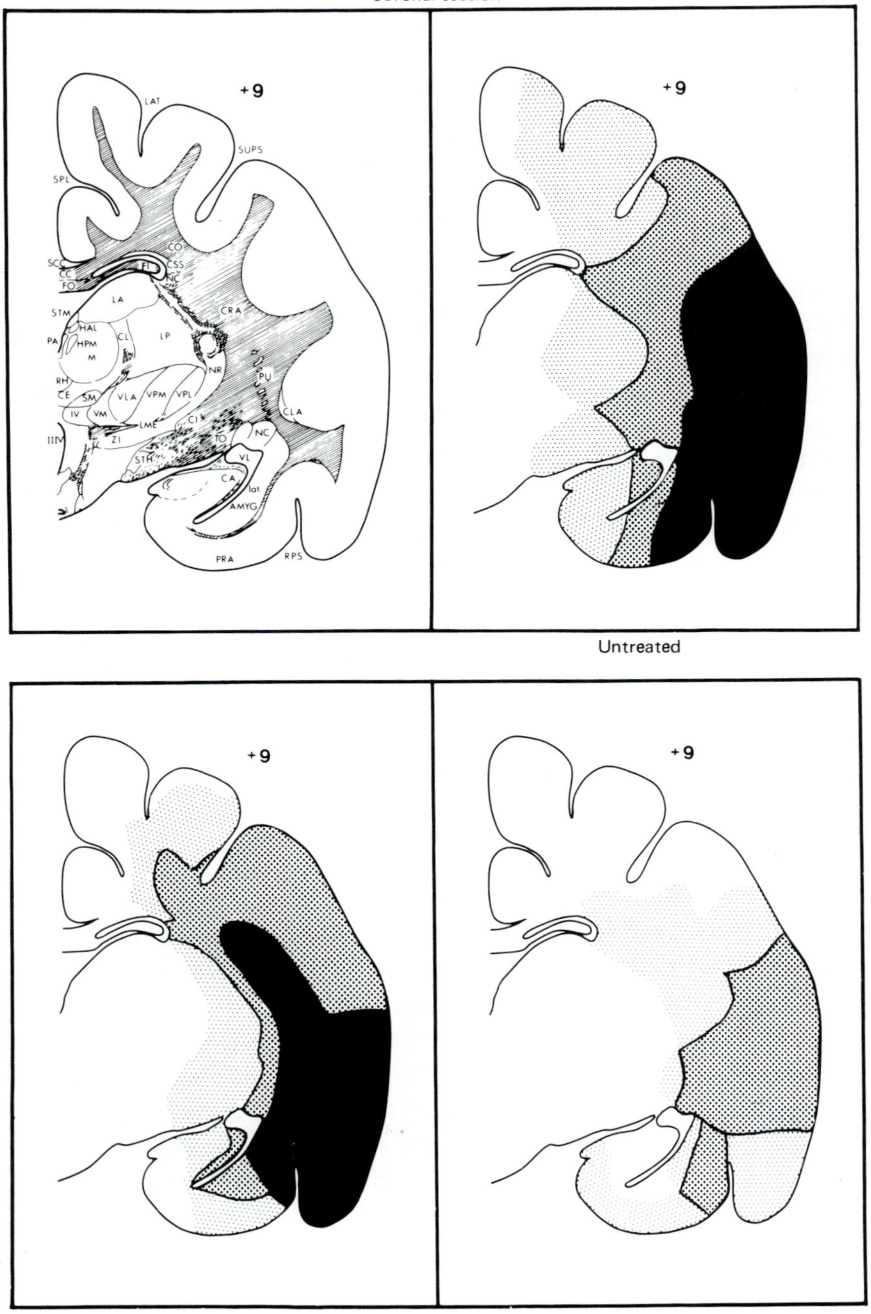

Untreated

1

Ifenprodil 5.6 µg/kg · min

Ifenprodil 16.7 µg/kg · min

Number of cats with necrotic lesions: 1–2; 3–4; ⩾5

(For legend, see p. 262.)

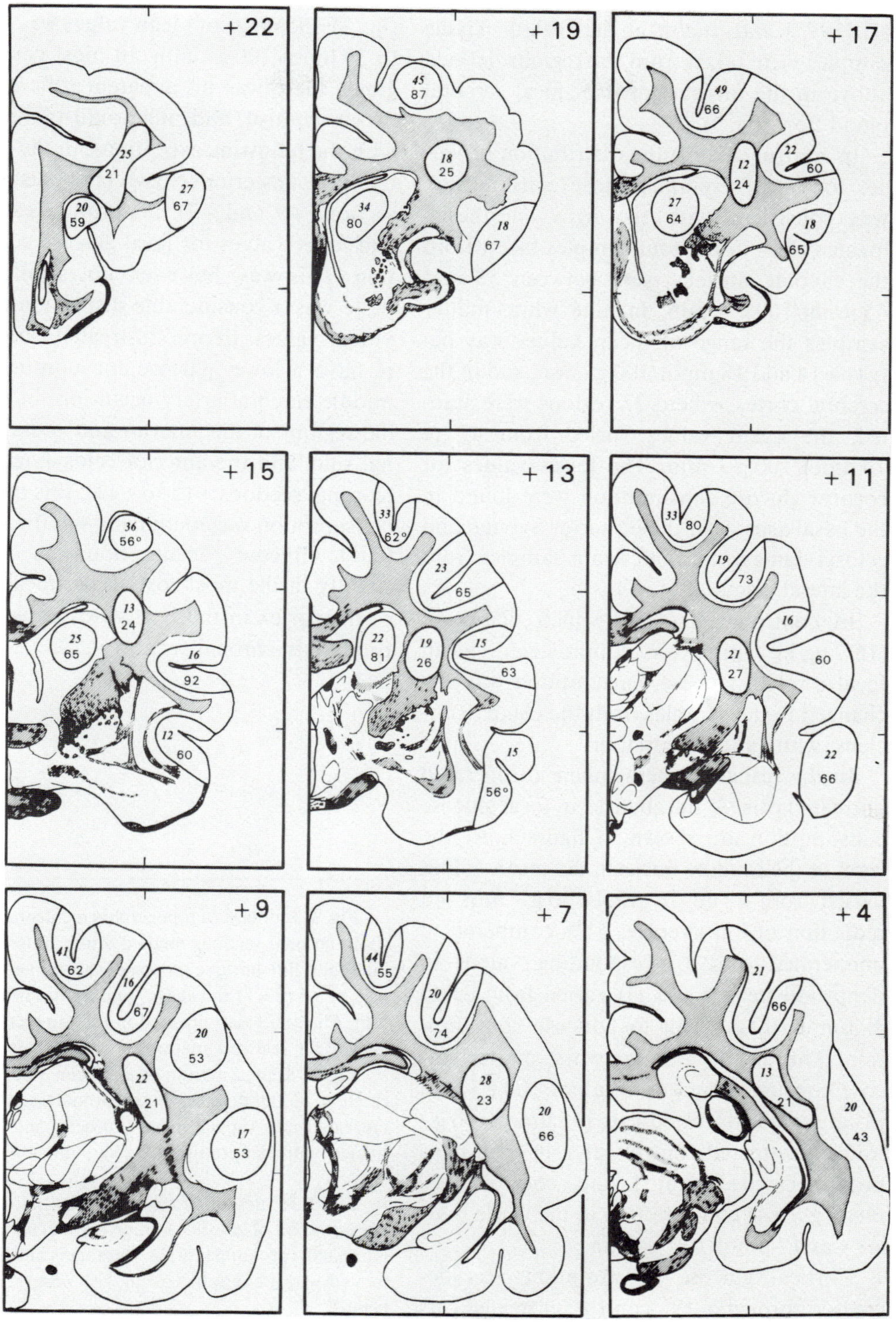

2

(For legend, see p. 262.)

al. [1977] and *Welsh* et al. [1980]. Tissue samples were taken from the regions defined above in the measurement of focal cerebral blood flow (fig. 3).

In control cats (4) the distribution of values for local cerebral glucose consumption was consistent with the light anesthesia: mean values in the four samples taken from the caudate nucleus were between 53 and 65 μmol/100 g · min; in nine white matter samples the range of mean values was between 14 and 18 μmol/100 g · min, and in the cerebral cortex, where 27 regions were studied, the mean values varied from 41 to 74 μmol/100 g · min. The lower values for cortical glucose consumption were found in the basal aspects of the posterior Sylvian and ectosylvian gyri and in certain samples from the lateral sulcus.

In control cats (4) to which ifenprodil (16.7 μg/kg · min) was administered, mean focal cerebral glucose consumption was unchanged in the samples from the caudate nucleus, white and grey matter.

In the ipsilateral hemisphere of operated untreated cats (3) the changes in focal glucose consumption are shown in figure 3. At the level of the caudate nucleus, the mean values varied from 22 to 36 μmol/100 g · min – a reduction of, on average, 51% compared to unoperated cats. Corresponding values in ifenprodil-treated cats (4) varied from 21 to 39 μmol/100 g · min for glucose consumption. The mean value for white matter glucose consumption was 18 μmol/100 g · min in untreated, operated cats (15 μmol/100 g · min in untreated control cats); in both ifenprodil-treated operated and control cats, mean glucose consumption in the white matter was 17 μmol/100 g · min.

Cortical glucose consumption was decreased throughout in control, untreated cats (fig. 3); the range of mean values was from 25 to 39 μmol/100 g · min. In most cortical regions, there was no apparent difference between control and ifenprodil-treated cats, with the following exceptions: in the convexity of the posterior ectosylvian gyrus (coronal sections +9 and +7), ifenprodil-treated cats had *lower* values for focal glucose consumption. This was, however, not significant as there was a considerable dispersion of individual values. Ifenprodil-treated cats tended to have a lower glucose consumption, after middle cerebral artery occlusion, in the caudal regions of the anterior and posterior rhinal sulci and the anterior ectosylvian sulcus (coronal sections +15 to +11); this decreased consumption was marginally significant ($p < 0.05$). Glucose consumption was increased slightly in the most rostral, perifocal regions of the cortex in those cats treated with ifenprodil (see coronal section +22).

Fig. 1. Montage of topographic incidence of necrosis in coronal sections studied 9 mm anterior to the interaural line in three groups of cats saline-treated (n = 6), at 5.6 (n = 7) and at 16.7 μg/kg · min ifenprodil (n = 6). The abbreviations used in the top section are to display the relevant anatomical structures.

Fig. 2. Representation of the mean values of local cerebral blood flow, at nine coronal sections, in 4 untreated cats (upper italic numbers) and in 4 cats treated with ifenprodil 5.6 μg/kg · min (lower numbers).

Fig. 3. Representation of the mean values of local consumption of glucose, at nine coronal sections, in 3 untreated cats (upper italic numbers) and in 4 cats treated with ifenprodil 16.7 μg/kg · min (lower numbers).

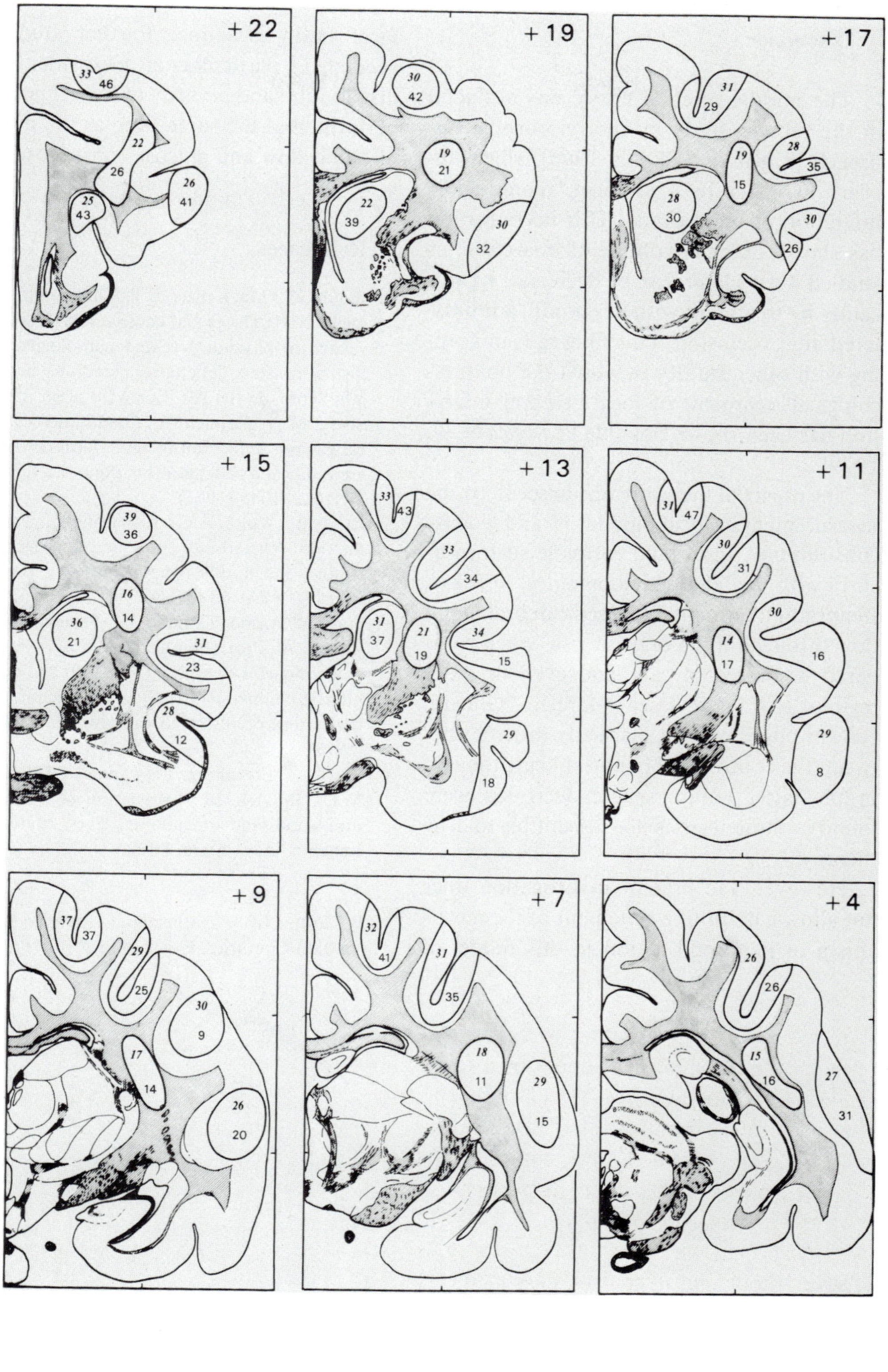
+22
33
46
22
26
26
41
25
43
+19
30
42
19
21
22
39
30
32
+17
31
29
19
15
28
35
28
30
30
26
+15
39
36
16
14
36
21
31
23
28
12
+13
33
43
33
34
31
37
21
19
34
15
29
18
+11
31
47
30
31
30
14
17
16
29
8
+9
37
37
29
25
30
9
17
14
26
20
+7
32
41
31
35
18
11
29
15
+4
26
26
15
16
27
31

3

Discussion

The middle cerebral artery was occluded in the present study by the retroorbital approach [*Sundt and Waltz,* 1966] which appears to result in a uniform, reproducible infarction of brain tissue. This investigation has shown that the volume of infarction, as studied 4 days later, can be decreased significantly by treatment with ifenprodil, administered after occlusion. This finding is in keeping with other studies in which the pharmacological treatment of focal cerebral infarction has been shown possible [*Tamura* et al., 1979].

The object of the study was to see if, by the measurement of focal blood flow and glucose consumption, one could correlate such measures with the later development of necrosis. Ifenprodil treatment increased cerebral blood flow throughout the brain at risk, when compared to untreated cats, and even in those regions that were later infarcted. Glucose consumption was not markedly different between the control and ifenprodil cats though, in the latter group, severe decreases were found in those regions *not* susceptible to drug therapy.

However, the present investigation does not allow a definitive statement of the mechanism of ifenprodil action in this model of focal brain ischemia. Further studies are needed; in particular, an assessment of the distribution and severity of ischemia changes performed at the same time as the measures of blood flow and glucose consumption.

References

Bartholini, G.; MacKenzie, E.T.; Depoortere, H.; Nowicki, J.-P.: Drugs and acute cerebral ischemia as related to physiological and pathological mechanisms; in Etats déficitaires cérébraux liés à l'âge. VIe Symp. de Bel Air, Evian (in press, 1980).

Ginsberg, M.D.; Reivich, R.; Giandomenico, A.: Local glucose utilization in acute focal cerebral ischemia. Local dysmetabolism. Neurology, Minneap. *27:* 1042–1048 (1977).

Sundt, T.M.; Waltz, A.G.: Experimental cerebral infarction: retroorbital, extradural approach for occluding the middle cerebral artery. Mayo Clin. Proc. *41:* 159–168 (1966).

Tamura, A.; Asano, T.; Sano, K.; Tsumagari, T.; Nakajima, A.: Protection from cerebral ischemia by a new imidazole derivative (Y-9179) and pentobarbital. A comparative study in chronic middle cerebral artery occlusion in cats. Stroke *10:* 126–134 (1979).

Welsh, F.A.; Greenberg, J.H.; Jones, S.C.; Ginsberg, M.D.; Reivich, M.: Correlation between glucose utilization and metabolite levels during focal ischemia in cat brain. Stroke *11:* 79–84 (1980).

B. Gotti, LERS, Synthelabo, 31, avenue Paul-Vaillant-Couturier, F–92220 Bagneux (France)

Eur. Neurol. *20:* 265–269 (1981)

Short-Term Memory and Cerebral Ischemia: Pharmacological Application

M. Le Poncin-Lafitte, C. Grosdemouge, C. Roy-Billon, D. Duterte, P. Potrat, P. Lespinasse, J.R. Rapin

Neurophysiologie cérébrovasculaire, CHU St-Antoine, Paris, France

Key Words. Avoidance response · Short-term memory · Cerebral blood flow · Cerebral metabolism · Edema

Abstract. Transient ischemia results in changes in the cerebral blood flow at the level of microinfarcts, enzymatic and metabolic changes and the development of a cerebral edema; all these disorders regress in the week following ischemia. Besides, the observed functional disorders disappear as the cerebral edema regresses. The brain functional activity is protected by the use of treatments which reduce the development of the cerebral edema and/or a quicker regression of the edema.

It is possible to reproduce a cerebral ischemia by using cerebral models for microembolism [3, 11]. The use of radioactive microspheres as an embolizing agent allows to determine the number of microspheres and their localization in the cerebral tissue [1]. Microembolization locally results in microinfarcts at the level of which a decrease in cerebral blood flow, metabolic and enzymatic changes [4] (fig. 1) and, secondarily, an edema are observed. These changes are to be related to the deterioration of the expression of short-term memory [10]. All these disorders disappear within 5 days and the edema regresses simultaneously: a transient ischemia with rapidly regressing sequelae was performed. We wanted to know whether, in these ischemic conditions, molecules influencing the development of the cerebral edema would also act on the functional sequelae induced by the cerebral ischemia.

Materials and Methods

Naive Long-Evans rats were exposed to a modified pole climbing test [2]; they were tested 10 times a day for 5 days [5]. Kinetics of the performance obtained during the conditioning session is reflected in an exponential curve [6]. After the last test session (day 5), the animals had acquired the avoidance response and they were exposed to an unilateral ischemia.

The animals were anaesthetized with chloral (360 mg/kg i.p.). 2,000 microspheres labelled with

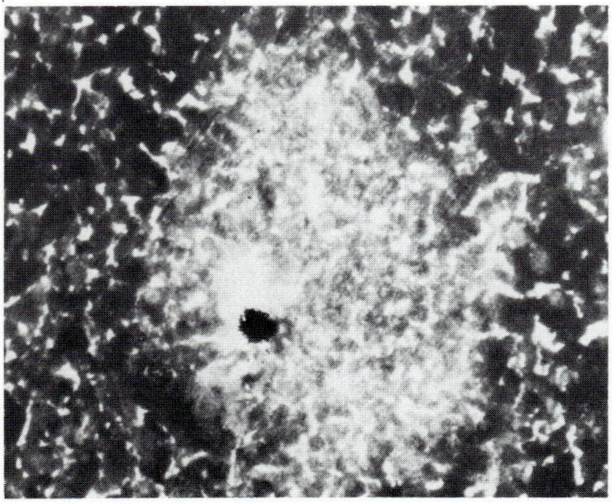

Fig. 1. Activity of NADH diaphorase. A shaded cone may be observed around the microsphere; it reflects the decrease in the enzymatic activity in the ischemized zone.

strontium-85 (⌀ 50 μ) were injected into the internal carotid which was ligated [10]; ischemia was performed in the right or in the left side, according to the functional predominance of the animal [8].

48 h later, the animals were again exposed to a conditioning session. In the last trial, cerebral blood flow, deoxyglucose uptake and consumption and edema were measured in the awaken animal during the conditioning session. Cerebral blood flow and deoxyglucose were simultaneously measured by means of an injection of iodoantipyrine labelled with iodine-125 and of deoxyglucose labelled with carbon-14 (25 μCi/rat) [9]. The extent of the brain edema was evaluated by assessing the brain water content.

Five groups of animals were formed: one control group and four groups of animals treated with either 200 μg/kg i.p. of nicergoline, 15 mg/kg i.p. of naftidrofuryl, 200 mg/kg of *Ginkgo biloba* per os or 100 mg/kg i.p. of cervilane.

Results

48 h after ischemia, the control group gave the escape response; the avoidance response was deteriorated. On the other hand the treated groups performed a satisfying avoidance response (fig. 2). 48 h after ischemia, there was a decrease in cerebral blood flow in the control group (fig. 3); this decrease in cerebral blood flow was not modified in the treated animals. 48 h after ischemia, there was a decrease in deoxyglucose uptake (fig. 4) and consumption (fig. 5a, b) in the control group; this effect of ischemia decreased in the treated animals. Evidently, in all treated groups the extent of edema was less important than in the control group (fig. 6).

Discussion

The number and localization of microspheres being known, quantitative microembolization allows to demonstrate the effects of ischemia not only at the hemodynamic and metabolic level but also at the functional level. Edema may be considered as a good index of the importance of embolization since there is a highly significant correlation between the development of edema and the number of microspheres localized in the nerve tissue [7]. The regression of edema in

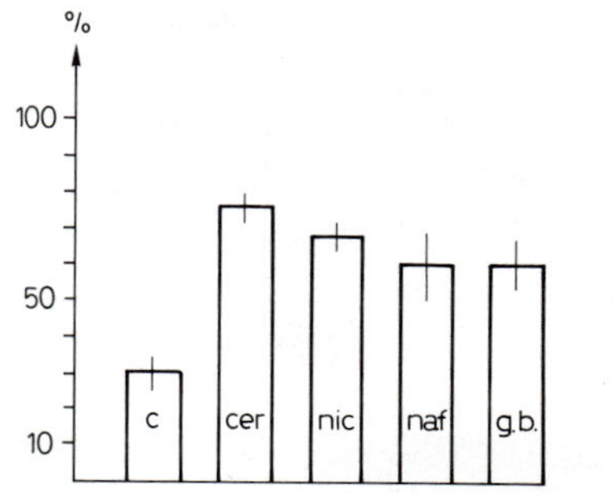

Fig. 2. Histogram of the performance level 48 h after ischemia (n = 10). Each value is a percentage mean value for the avoidance response ± SEM. c = Control group; cer = cervilane (100 mg/kg i.p.); nic = nicergoline (200 µg/kg i.p.); naf = naftidrofuryl (15 mg/kg); g.b. = *Ginkgo biloba* (200 mg/kg per os).

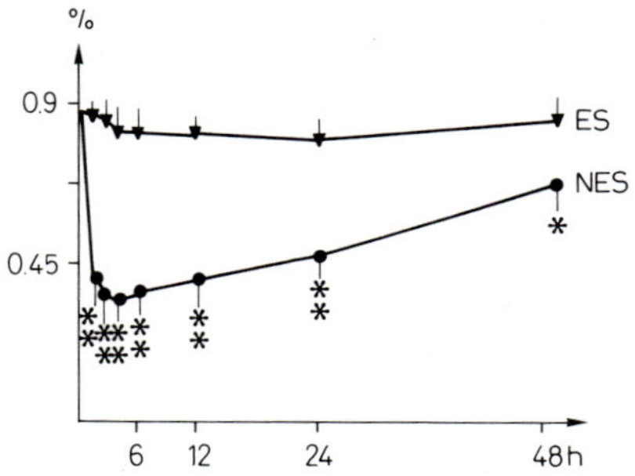

Fig. 3. Cerebral blood flow at various time intervals after ischemia in the awaken animals (ES = embolized side, NES = nonembolized side). On the ordinate, percentage of cardiac output in brain and on the abscissa, the various times after microembolization (2,000 microspheres into the internal carotid) are shown.

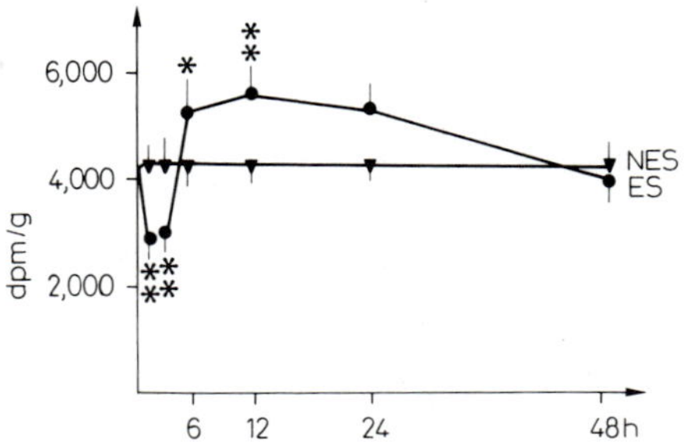

Fig. 4. Deoxyglucose uptake measures at various time intervals after ischemia in the awaken animals (n = 10; ES = embolized side; NES = nonembolized side).

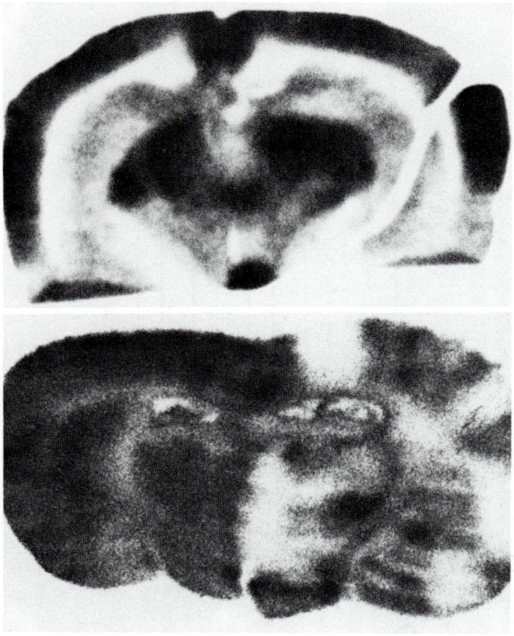

a

b

Fig. 5. Deoxyglucose consumption measure by autoradiographic method (Sokoloff technique) in the awaken animal. **a** Control animal. **b** Ischemized animal: autoradiographic method.

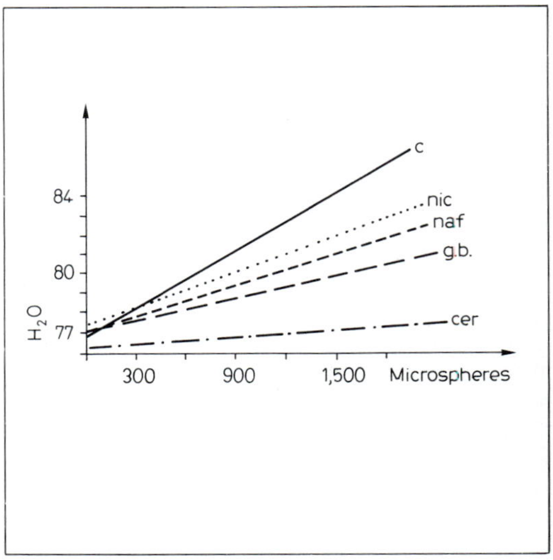

Fig. 6. Correlation between the cerebral edema (percentage of water) in control and treated animals and the number of microspheres. Control (c): y = 76.80 + 0.0049 x (r = 0.95); nicergoline (nic): y = 77.31 + 0.0024 x (r = 0.91); naftidrofuryl (naf): y = 76.96 + 0.0019 x (r = 0.81); *Ginkgo biloba* (g.b.): y = 77.20 + 0.0021 x (r = 0.83); cervilane (cer): y = 76.30 + 0.0017 x (r = 0.81).

the 5 days following ischemia is to be related to the cell metabolism recovery and certainly to a new vascularization of the ischemized zone. Besides, we previously showed that there was a perfect correlation between the regression of edema and the reappearing avoidance response and that the temporary loss of the avoidance response did not seem to be due to the disturbance of the mnemonic imprint but could be related to the compressions resulting from the edema in areas involved in the conditioned responses and/or the transmission pathways. When compressions are suppressed because of the regression of edema, the avoidance response reappears.

In this type of transient ischemia with rapidly regressing sequelae, it therefore seems necessary to prescribe a treatment allowing to reduce, if not suppress, the development of cerebral edema; in this work, we showed that molecules which allow a better recovery of the functional activity are also those influencing the development of edema which they reduce; their effect of the deoxyglucose capture and uptake is only secondarily.

The mechanism by which these molecules may reduce the extent of edema following this type of cerebral ischemia remains to be determined.

References

1 Bralet, A.M.; Rochette, L.; Rapin, J.R.; Bralet, J.: Localisation et effets à court terme d'une embolisation cérébrale réalisée chez le rat par injection intracarotidienne de microsphères. J. Pharmacol., Paris *8:* 241 (1977).

2 Courvoisier, S.J.; Fournel, R.; Ducrot, R.; Kolsky, M.; Koetschet, P.: Propriétés pharmacologiques du chlorhydrate de chloro-3-(diméthyl-amino-3-propyl)-10-phenothiazine (4560 R.P.). Archs int. Pharmacodyn. Thér. *92:* 305–361 (1953).

3 Kogure, K.; Busto, R.; Scheinberg, P.; Reinuth, O.M.: Energy metabolism and water content in rat brain during the early stage of development of cerebral infarction. Brain *97:* 103–114 (1974).

4 Lageron, A.; Le Poncin-Lafitte, M.; Rapin, J.R.: Brain rat histoenzymological changes induced by microsphere injection during ischemia. Acta histochem. *65:* 184–190 (1979).

5 Le Poncin, M.; Charpentier, J.: Effets de la fumée de tabac par voie respiratoire sur le conditionnement d'évitement chez le rat. J. Physiol., Paris *65:* 444 (1972).

6 Le Poncin-Lafitte, M.; Pesquies, P.C.; Lafitte, J.C.; Rapin, J.R.: Détermination des paramètres cinétiques d'un conditionnement: applications expérimentales et validité de l'étude. J. Pharmacol., Paris *10:* 262 (1979).

7 Le Poncin-Lafitte, M.; Rapin, J.; Rapin, J.R.: Effects of *Ginkgo biloba* on changes induced by quantitative ischemia microembolization in rats. Archs int. Pharmacodyn. Thér. *243:* 244–263 (1980).

8 Le Poncin-Lafitte, M.; Rapin, J.R.: Preuve de la latéralisation hémisphérique fonctionnelle chez le rat. J. Physiol., Paris (in press, 1980).

9 Le Poncin-Lafitte, M.; Rapin, J.; Rapin, J.R.: Effects of an extract of *Ginkgo biloba* on the cerebral changes induced by a quantitative ischemia; in Betz et al., Pathophysiology and pharmacotherapy of cerebrovascular disorders, pp. 277–280 (Witzstrock, Baden-Baden 1980).

10 Le Poncin-Lafitte, M.; Roy-Billon, C.; Duterte, D.; Grosdemouge, C.; Rapin, J.R.: Effects of quantitative cerebral microembolisms on microcirculation and learning in Long-Evans rats. Cerebral microcirculation and metabolism (Raven Press, New York, in press 1980).

11 Meyer, J.S.; Gotoh, F.; Tazaki, Y.: Circulation and metabolism following experimental embolism. J. Neuropath. exp. Neurol. *21:* 4–24 (1962).

M. Le Poncin-Lafitte, Cerebrovascular Neurophysiology Department, CHU St-Antoine, 27, rue de Chaligny, F–75012 Paris (France)

Eur. Neurol. *20:* 270–272 (1981)

Determination of Regional Cerebral Glucose Transport and Utilization Rates in Man with ^{11}C-Glucose: Preliminary Results[1]

J.C. Depresseux, A. Feron, J.M. Peters, G. Del Fiore, L. Quaglia

Cyclotron Research Center, University of Liège, Belgium

Key Words. Brain · ^{11}C-Glucose · Model

Abstract. This paper describes the methodology and the first results of a method of measurement of the cerebral metabolic rate of glucose, using ^{11}C-glucose and regional detection by probes. The present method has the advantages of being rapidly repeatable and of yielding a determination of the rates of transfer of glucose across the blood-brain barrier.

Introduction

The measurement of the regional cerebral blood flow with diffusible inert gases or non-diffusible tracers brought the hope of many potentials of progress in the understanding of cerebral circulation and function in man. Theses approaches nevertheless encounter several limitations, particularly in the interpretation of physiopathological phenomena – such as the luxury perfusion syndrome – and in the implementation of useful clinical applications.

The difficulty results mainly from the lack of non-invasive and reliable methods for the study of the cerebral metabolism in man.

The nervous and glial cells are restricted almost exclusively to glucose as the substrate for their energy metabolism. The measurement of the rate of cerebral uptake of glucose appears therefore as a valuable approach to the study of the energy supply and utilization in the various regions of the brain.

Method

Glucose randomly labeled with carbon-11 is prepared in our laboratory by photosynthesis, using Chlorella algae rather than green leaves [1]. This original method of labeling has the advantage of yielding very high and reliable levels of activity of ^{11}C-*d*-glucose.

After radiochemical and radiopharmaceutical controls, 7 mCi of ^{11}C-*d*-glucose are injected intravenously. The regional transfer functions in the brain are detected and registered during the 3 min following the injection, by means of a multiprobe device with shields and collimators allowing the simultaneous study of up to 26 distinct cerebral area.

1 Supported by a grant from the National Foundation for Scientific Research.

Table I. The main parameters ruling the transport and utilization of glucose in the brain computed with the ^{11}C-glucose method

Φ_{43}	cerebral metabolic rate of glucose	26.2	μmol glucose [100 g tissue]$^{-1}$ min^{-1}
Φ_{32}	forward flux of glucose through the BBB	87.2	μmol glucose [100 g tissue]$^{-1}$ min^{-1}
Φ_{23}	reverse flux of glucose through the BBB	61.0	μmol glucose [100 g tissue]$^{-1}$ min^{-1}
Q_vW^{-1}	intravascular free glucose mass	21.2	μmol glucose [100 g tissue]$^{-1}$
Q_3W^{-1}	extravascular free glucose mass	132.0	μmol glucose [100 g tissue]$^{-1}$
C_3/C_v	brain-to-blood concentration ratio	0.529	

Values obtained in a normal subject are displayed. BBB = Blood-brain barrier.

The model of interpretation of the data and their numerical analysis are based on the previous experiments performed on monkeys by *Raichle* et al. [2, 3].

The unlabeled and labeled glucose are considered to be distributed through four subsystems, in each detected area of head: subsystem 1, the intravascular inexchangeable glucose in the arteries and veins; subsystem 2, the intravascular exchangeable glucose in the capillaries; subsystem 3, the extravascular unmetabolized glucose; subsystem 4, the metabolites of glucose.

Three main assumptions are at the basis of the mathematical formulation of the model.

(1) The transport and metabolism of labeled glucose are assumed to be ruled by the same dynamic constants as the substrate under study. In the present method, this assumption is valid, because of the biochemical identity between the tracer and the traced compound.

(2) The flow rate and concentrations of glucose through the system are assumed to be in a steady state during the time interval (3 min) of measurements.

(3) The outflow of ^{11}C-labeled metabolites of glucose is assumed to be negligeable between the injection time and the end of detection of the transfer function of glucose in the head. This point has been controlled and validated by *Raichle* et al. [2, 3].

The mathematical development of the model yields an equation with three parameters and two variables:

$$\chi = \frac{r_{hg}(T) - r_{vg}(T)}{\frac{\alpha}{\alpha - 1}\int_O^T r_{vg}(t)dt - \frac{\kappa}{\alpha - 1}\int_O^T e^{-\kappa t}\, r_{vg}(t)dt}.$$

The three parameters are as follows: χ is the ratio between the net flux of glucose to the tissues and the intravascular mass of glucose; α is the ratio between forward and reverse fluxes of glucose through the blood-brain barrier, and κ is the sum of the transport constants of glucose out of compartment 3.

The formula contains also two time-dependent variables: r_{hg} is the value of the transfer function of labeled glucose through the detection field, and r_{vg} is the corresponding value in the intravascular compartment.

The values of the variable r_{vg} are not measured directly but are computed from a second set of data, obtained after intravenous injection of ^{11}CO-tagged red blood cells.

The detection data obtained with the head probes and with an additional probe detecting the activity in an arterial catheter, after injection of ^{11}C-glucose and of ^{11}CO-erythrocytes, allow us to compute the function r_{vg}, with the aid of a convolution-deconvolution procedure.

Results

The results are displayed in two ways: (1) as an analytical display of the transfer functions of ^{11}C through the intravascular glucose, extravascular glucose and glucose metabolites compartments, and (2) as a table of derived parameters, particularly, the cerebral metabolic rate of glucose, and the parameters ruling the transport of glucose through the blood-brain barrier, namely the glucose tissular concentration and space of diffusion and, also, the forward and reverse fluxes of glucose through the barrier (table I).

The results, obtained in the normal human at rest, are consistent with the values computed for the whole normal brain from the data obtained by *Reivich* et al. [4] using ^{18}F-fluorodeoxyglucose as a tracer.

Conclusion

These results are preliminary, but even now the attractiveness of the present method lies in its applicability to human studies, in its repeatability, in its potentiality for regional studies and, finally, in the possibility of assessing not only the uptake rate of glucose, but also the transport of this substrate through the blood-brain barrier. It appears to us that the possible alterations of this transport are not to be overlooked, especially in pathological cases and in pharmacological studies, and that the present method brings a valuable tool for research in the metabolism of the brain.

References

1 Feron, A.; Peters, J.M.; Del Fiore, G.; Quaglia, L.; Depresseux, J.C.; Bartsch, P.: Photosynthesis of ^{11}C-labeled glucose with algae. Eur. J. nucl. Med. 5A. *17* (1980).

2 Raichle, M.E.; Larson, K.B.; Phelps, M.E.; Grubb, R.L.; Walch, M.J.; Ter-Pogossian, M.M.: In vivo measurement of brain glucose transport and metabolism employing glucose ^{11}C. Am. J. Physiol. *228:* 1936–1948 (1975).

3 Raichle, M.E.; Welch, M.J.; Grubb, R.L.; Higgins, C.G.; Ter-Pogossian, M.M.; Larson, K.B.: Measurement of regional substrate utilization rates by emission tomography. Science *199:* 986–987 (1978).

4 Reivich, R.; Kuhl, D.; Wolf, A.; Greenberg, J.; Phelps, M.; Ido, I.; Casella, V.; Fowler, J.; Hoffman, E.; Alavi, A.; Som, P.; Sokoloff, L.: The ^{18}F fluoro deoxyglucose method for the measurement of local cerebral glucose utilization in man. Circulation Res. *44:* 127–137 (1979).

J.C. Depresseux, Cyclotron Research Center,
University of Liège, Liège (Belgium)

Eur. Neurol. *20:* 273–284 (1981)

Noninvasive Tomographic Study of Cerebral Blood Flow and Oxygen Metabolism in vivo

Potentials, Limitations, and Clinical Applications in Cerebral Ischemic Disorders

J.C. Baron, M.G. Bousser, D. Comar, F. Soussaline, P. Castaigne

Commissariat à l'Energie Atomique, Service Hospitalier Frédéric-Joliot, Orsay, France; Clinique des Maladies du Système Nerveux, La Salpêtrière, Paris, France

Key Words. Cerebral blood flow · Cerebral oxygen metabolism · Positron emission tomography · Cerebral ischemia · ^{15}O inhalation

Abstract. The non-invasive continuous inhalation technique of $C^{15}O_2$ and $^{15}O_2$ coupled with positron emission tomography (PET) provides brain images that are thought to represent local cerebral blood flow (CBF) and oxygen extraction fraction (OEF). Experimental studies in baboons have confirmed that $C^{15}O_2$ inhalation allows tomographic measurement of CBF. The numerous difficulties involved in PET absolute quantitation are stressed, as well as some limitations inherent to the ^{15}O inhalation model. However, the values for local CBF, OEF and $CMRO_2$ obtained in normal young subjects are satisfactory in view of the above-mentioned limitations.

The clinical application to recent cerebral infarction has allowed two opposite types of flow-metabolism uncoupling to be identified, which appear to be often predictive of tissue prognosis. The time course of spontaneous changes in CBF and OEF within the infarct is also described. Our studies have, in addition, revealed the previously unknown phenomenon of 'crossed cerebellar diaschisis' in supratentorial infarction. Lastly, a state of chronic watershed ischemia, potentially reversible by surgical revascularization, has been identified as presumably involved in the progression of watershed necrosis. The clinical potentials of this method appear considerable.

Introduction

Despite considerable improvement in the prevention of cerebral ischemic disorder during the last few decades, no significant therapeutic progress has yet been achieved in the management of patients with completed ischemic stroke. However, a better understanding of the pathophysiologic phenomena underlying the cerebral ischemic process may lead to differentiate tissue irreparably condemned to necrosis from tissue which might recover its function following a logically adapted therapeutic action.

In such research, the development of various methods for measuring in man the regional cerebral blood flow (CBF) and, in a much smaller scale, the regional metabolism, have yielded a wealth of essential information [16]. However, most techniques have been limited because they are either invasive, or poorly regional, or do not provide regional measurement of metabolic parameters. The latter are especially crucial in cerebrovascular disease because of the recognized frequency of situations where blood flow and metabolism are uncoupled; it is, then, difficult to draw much relevant information about the functional state of the brain tissue when perfusion is the only parameter investigated.

The recent development of positron emission tomography (PET) [39] is theoretically capable of considerably changing research on the pathophysiology of cerebral ischemia in man. It becomes now possible to noninvasively obtain quantified tomographic images of high spatial resolution that map not only CBF, but also oxygen and glucose consumption, cerebral blood volume, and many other parameters [33]. It is, in fact, close to an 'in vivo autoradiography' [33] in man.

Among the PET techniques for imaging CBF and metabolism, we chose the ^{15}O continuous inhalation technique [23] because it is particularly well suited to the study of cerebral ischemic disorders. For this purpose, the other PET techniques have major disadvantages. Combined imaging of CBF and glucose consumption by respective intravenous injection of $^{13}NH_3$ and ^{18}F-2-deoxy-glucose, used by some in studying cerebral infarction [25], is apparently valid only in healthy brain, since, in both instances, tracer behavior in diseased brain remains unpredictable at our present state of knowledge [18, 30]. Moreover, functional assessement of ischemic-anoxic brain by measurement of glucose consumption may be highly controversial since anaerobic glycolysis may then be at play. The technique using ^{77}Kr [44] by single inhalation is intrinsically limited by the very fact that it only measures CBF. The ^{15}O continuous inhalation technique, on the contrary, is the only presently available technique that allows tomographic measurement of CBF and oxygen metabolism, and its validity should be essentially preserved in the ischemic brain. A dynamic PET technique for measuring regional oxygen and glucose consumption by respective single inhalation of $^{15}O_2$ and intravenous of ^{11}C-glucose has been recently proposed [34], but the technological difficulties involved appear, as yet, serious.

Principle and Methods

They have been described in detail elsewhere [5], and will only be briefly summarized here.

The patient continuously inhales to equilibrium trace amounts of $C^{15}O_2$ and $^{15}O_2$ consecutively, which are delivered at both constant rate and concentration from a medical cyclotron. Axial transverse tomographic images (thickness: 2 cm; lateral resolution: 1.5 cm) of cerebral radioactive distribution are collected at identical levels using a positron tomograph (model ECAT, ORTEC), the characteristics of which have previously been described [31, 36]. Because of the very short half-life of the tracer, a state of 'dynamic equilibrium' is reached after 6–10 days of continuous inhalation so that blood and tissue radioactive concentrations are stable: the constant input of radioactivity is equal to its disappearance by radioactive decay and physiological transport. The theoretical model [23] states that, because of the total and immediate transfer of the tracer to blood water, the continuous inhalation of $C^{15}O_2$ in fact labels in vivo the water of the body, and the cerebral concentration of $H_2{}^{15}O$ is then proportional to blood flow. This relation is, however, nonlinear so that for high blood flows, the increase in radioactivity is much smaller than the real increase in CBF. Inhalation of $^{15}O_2$ labels in vivo hemoglobin ($Hb^{15}O_2$) and the tissues take up the tracer in proportion to their oxygen consumption rate and immediately combine it with hydrogen from respiration to locally form labelled water ($H_2{}^{15}O$). The latter is, however, constantly cleared by effluent flow, which leads to the recirculation of the $H_2{}^{15}O$. The cerebral distribution of equilibrium $H_2{}^{15}O$ during inhalation of $^{15}O_2$ will consequently be proportional to both oxygen consumption ($CMRO_2$) and CBF. The theoretical model indicates, however, that the division, pixel by pixel, of the $^{15}O_2$ image by the corresponding $C^{15}O_2$ image eliminates the CBF component and provides a ratio image the distribution of which is linearly proportional to the oxygen extraction fraction [OEF = (Ca – Cv)/(Ca), where Ca and Cv are, respectively, the arterial and venous oxygen contents]. For each cerebral level studied, a set of three tomographic images are obtained: $C^{15}O_2$ (representing CBF), $^{15}O_2$ (both $CMRO_2$ and CBF) and $^{15}O_2/C^{15}O_2$ (ratio representing OEF).

PET Absolute Quantitation of CBF, OEF and $CMRO_2$

Absolute quantitation of regional CBF, OEF and $CMRO_2$ using the ^{15}O continuous inhalation technique coupled with PET is theoretically feasible using a simple mathematical model developed by *Jones* et al. [23], and later refined by *Subramanyam* et al. [37] and *Lenzy* et al. [27]. This quantitation would be highly desirable because the $C^{15}O_2$ and the $^{15}O_2/C^{15}O_2$ ratio qualitative images are only relative representations of CBF and OEF, respectively, from which no accurate assessment of regional $CMRO_2$ can be derived. Conversely, if the quantitative values obtained in control studies of normal subjects were comparable to known normal values, this would heavily support the validity of both the principle and the mathematical model that describe the ^{15}O continuous inhalation technique.

Among the few steps necessary to obtain such quantitative data, the most important one is the accurate absolute measurement of the equilibrium radioactive concentrations in both the cerebral region of interest and the peripheral arterial blood (the latter can be obtained by femoral puncture and is reasonably equated to the cerebral arterial-capillary tracer concentration). Another necessary but straightforward measurement is that of the arterial oxygen content.

Practically, however, this involves several technological difficulties. Stable equilibrium can be easily obtained, provided the rate of delivery of the radioactive gas is held constant and the patient is cooperative enough. Accurate measurement of arterial $H_2{}^{15}O$ and $Hb^{15}O_2$ concentrations has not, in our experience, been a major difficulty [6]. A considerably more difficult task is that of accurately measuring regional cerebral $H_2{}^{15}O$ concentration. It must be emphasized that this is not specific to the ^{15}O technique, but rather is a challenge that applies to any brain study with PET. Although it has been amply demonstrated that PET quantitative measurements can be satisfactorily accurate ($\sim \pm 5\%$) when imaging a cylindrical phantom filled with a radioactive solution of known concentration [31, 36], major problems arise when one considers the human head. (In this respect, it must be recalled that the published values for regional glucose consumption using ^{18}F-2-deoxy-glucose and either single photon [35] or positron emission tomography [32] in normal as well as in diseased brain have been derived empirically since the so-called 'lumped-constant' for fluorodeoxyglucose has, as yet, never been directly measured neither in man nor in the animal [32].) Unlike the phantom, the head is quite heterogenous in respect to its gamma-ray attenuation coefficient (scalp, skull and brain have different absorption coefficients), so that mathematically applying a uniform absorption coefficient potentially leads to serious errors in the reconstructed regional radioactive concentrations [22]. However, this difficulty can be accurately overcome by applying to the original scan an accurate attenuation correction by means of a transmission scan performed at the same brain level, although this procedure decreases the signal-to-noise ratio in the final image. As with any quantitative study using radionuclides, it is essential to carry out as accurately and as frequently as possible a system calibration relative to the wall-counter taking into account the geometry of the organ of interest, i.e., a head-sized phantom in the present case. Another feature of the in vivo situation is the anatomical and physiological complexity of the brain: given the above-mentioned spatial resolution of the ECAT system in standard clinical conditions, many if not all cerebral structures are of insufficient sizes to be faithfully imaged; particularly, no area consisting uniquely of pure gray or pure white matter is available. Phantom studies have shown that an object must have a diameter at least twice the system spatial resolution (i.e. approximately 3 cm) if the total amount of radioactivity contained within its limits is to be recovered [19]. Moreover, radioactive heterogeneities within the brain results in a heterogenous Compton scatter leading to further contrast degradation. Other less serious problems are the random coincidences (that can be subtracted on line), the variation of slice thickness across the field of view (axial resolution), and the fact that brain is both irregularly shaped (noncylindrical object) and constituted of parenchymal as well as nonparenchymal (blood vessels, ventricules, etc.) structures. Obviously, while many of the above difficulties can be largely minimized by taking appropriate precautions, others cannot be overcome and simply have to be taken into account when interpreting the PET data.

The first attempts to quantify CBF, OEF and $CMRO_2$ using the ECAT system were relatively unsatisfactory [6] and conflicted with results obtained by others using a different PET system [3]. This raised questions concerning the validity of the ^{15}O continuous inhalation model, for which only indirect evidence was available [2]. However, a better understanding of the above-mentioned technological difficulties led to designing an experimental study in baboons, using the well-known relationship between CBF and $PaCO_2$, that clearly demonstrated that $C^{15}O_2$ continuous inhalation allows tomographic measurement of CBF [9]. During the course of this study, a point was raised concerning the consequences of the nonlinearity of the tissue $H_2{}^{15}O$-CBF relationship. In this regard, the inescapable admixture of two components with different blood flows and water partition coefficients – namely, gray and white matter –, whatever the size and location of the region under consideration, results in systematic underestimation of the computed CBF by as much as 25%. This latter effect can be minimized by choosing very small regions of interest in selected areas thought to contain the highest possible proportion of, respectively, gray and white matter [17].

Using this procedure, the measured regional CBF, OEF and $CMRO_2$ in a limited number of healthy young subjects compare quite well with generally accepted normal values (fig. 1). How a similar procedure can be extended to diseased brain has not yet been fully worked out.

Other potential errors of secondary importance are: (1) the alleged limitation in brain water permeability [15] that would induce underestimation of the computed gray CBF; (2) the uncertainties concerning the re-

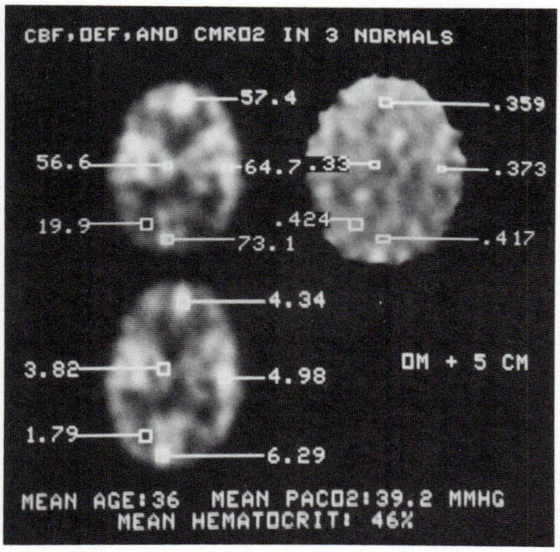

Fig. 1. Local CBF (upper left), OEF (upper right) and $CMRO_2$ (lower left) images in a normal subject. The regional values indicated are the mean of the 3 normals for small regions of interest not necessarily located in the same area in all 3 subjects, but selected in each in order to have the highest possible proportion of gray or, when appropriate, white matter. The range of CBF, OEF and $CMRO_2$ for predominantly gray matter are 56.6–73.1cm^3/100 g/min, 0.33–0.42, and 3.82–6.29 ml O_2/100 g/min, respectively. White matter values are 19.9, 0.424 and 1.79 for CBF, OEF and $CMRO_2$, respectively.

spective densities of the various brain structures and of blood; (3) the presence of radioactive blood within brain parenchyma that induces overestimation of both measured CBF and OEF, and (4) the tissue content of dissolved oxygen increasing the computed OEF value.

Lastly, because the $C^{15}O_2$ model is sensitive to measurement errors at high flow rates as a result of its nonlinearity, the precision of the CBF measurement has been estimated by some, on theoretical bases, to be unacceptably poor [21]. Our baboons studies have shown, however, the measurement reproducibility of regional CBF to be ± (SD) 10.4%, a satisfactory value when one considers all the potential measurement errors on top of the expected physiological variability [9].

In summary, both the overall validity of the ^{15}O inhalation model and the feasibility of PET absolute quantitation of CBF, OEF and $CMRO_2$ have been demonstrated. This technique does have – like any physiological measurement – some limitations, but it obviously has tremendous clinical potentials. The latter will be fully exploited when, in the very near future, the quantitation of local CBF, OEF and $CMRO_2$ in any given region, whether in normal or in diseased brain, has been fully worked out.

Clinical Application in the Pathophysiologic Study of Cerebral Ischemic Disorders

Because of the above-mentioned difficulties, both theoretical and practical, that are involved in absolute quantitation of CBF, OEF and $CMRO_2$ using the ^{15}O inhalation technique, our experience of quantitation in patients is limited, and only semiquantitative data will be reported. On the images obtained, count rates per unit volume were computed for various regions of interest, and compared to the values obtained from contralateral homologous regions; the side-to-side difference was considered abnormal if it lay outside the confidence limits defined for roughly similar regions in 17 control studies. Thus, when desirable, a percent index of asymmetry in both CBF ($C^{15}O_2$ image) and OEF ($^{15}O_2/C^{15}O_2$ ratio image) could be obtained in any brain area.

As can be seen in figure 1, the normal brain is characterized by the close similarity between the CBF and $CMRO_2$ images; in other words, the OEF is essentially constant throughout all brain structures. This describes the normal couple between CBF and oxygen metabolism, the former being tightly adjusted to the latter by a constant relationship.

55 patients suffering from complete ischemic stroke were studied, 7 of whom were studied twice. 50 patients had a single infarct, 4 patients had two, and 1 patient had three infarcts. A total of 68 supratentorial infarcts, the age from onset of which varied between 30 h and 20 years, were consequently studied. Diagnosis was clinically established and confirmed by ancillary diagnostic procedures (including CT scan in 32 patients) or by postmortem study in 2 patients. Of the 68 infarcts, 53 were in the area of the middle cerebral artery (MCA), 9 in that of the posterior cerebral artery, and 6 were classified as watershed infarcts. Preliminary findings have already been published [7, 8].

Within the first few weeks following the clinical onset, a state of focal disruption of the normal flow-metabolism couple, as evidenced by a focal OEF anomaly, has been observed in the vast majority of the cases studied. Out of 45 infarcts dating less than 31 days, there were 43 (95%) instances where the OEF was focally disturbed, even though in several cases this was restricted to only part of the entire zone where either or both CBF and OEF were impaired in a heterogenous pattern. Two radically opposite types of uncoupling have been observed.

The first of these two types of uncoupling is characterized by a *decrease* in OEF (fig. 4), consequently implying a focal decrease of the arteriovenous oxygen difference: this meets the criteria defining *Lassen*'s 'luxury-perfusion syndrome' [26]. We observed the phenomenon in 37 of 45 (82%) infarcts dating less than 31 days. The area showing 'luxury-perfusion' i.e. decreased OEF, displayed decreased CBF in 52% of the cases, normal flow in 34% and focal hyperemia in 14% of the cases. Thus, even though perfusion is normal or even decreased, it is still overabundant relative to the metabolic needs of the brain tissue, the corollary being a decrease in the oxygen arteriovenous difference. However, since for many years only CBF measurements were available, the notion of 'luxury-perfusion' in cerebral infarction was equated to focal hyperemia only [16]. The possibility opened by the ^{15}O inhalation technique coupled with PET, of imaging both perfusion and oxygen metabolism now demonstrates that most, if not all, recent infarcts go through a phase where the 'luxury-perfusion syndrome' is prominent, whether associated with normal, decreased or increased flow, as suggested by previous experimental stroke studies [42].

The second type of disruption of the flow-metabolism couple is characterized by an OEF focal *increase*. We observed this in 9 of 45 (18%) recent infarcts, constantly associated with decreased perfusion. Such oxygen fractional hyperextraction indicates that perfusion is now insufficient to meet the metabolic requirements of the tissue. Because it involves a state diametrically contrary to 'luxury-perfusion', it has been jocularly termed the 'misery-perfusion syndrome' [8]. In 4 of the above-mentioned 9 cases, the two states coexist in adjacent regions. Focal oxygen fractional hyperextraction has been reported by other users of the ^{15}O inhalation method [1, 40]. Similarly, in experimental occlusion of the MCA in the animal, a transient darkening of the venous blood draining the cortical area subject to acute ischemia, i.e.

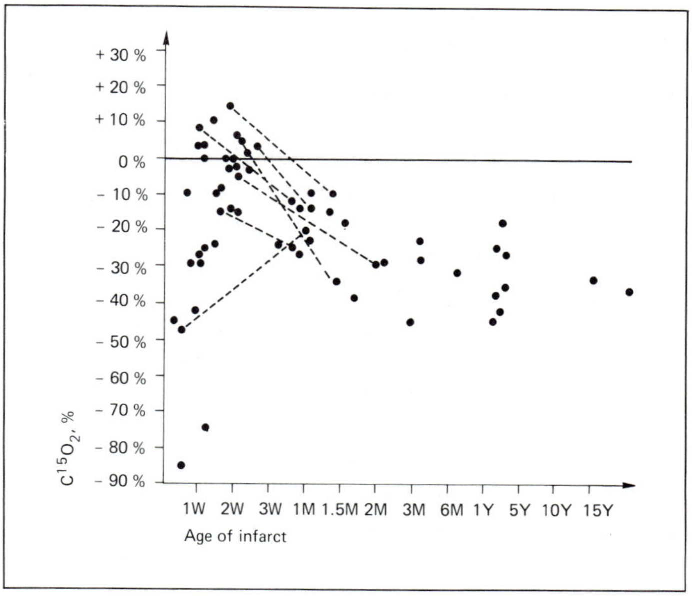

Fig. 2. $C^{15}O_2$ count rate within the infarct relative to the unaffected side (contralateral homologous area), i.e. a percent reflection of the mean change in CBF in 62 infarcts as a function of age from onset. The broken lines represent 7 infarcts studied on two occasions (see text). W = Week; m = month; Y = year.

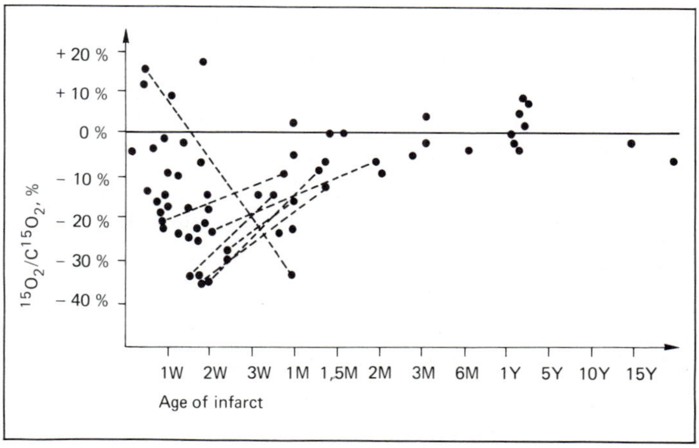

Fig. 3. $^{15}O_2/C^{15}O_2$ ratio count rate within the infarct relative to the unaffected side (contralateral homologous area), i.e., a reflection of the percent change in the OEF in the same 62 infarcts as shown in figure 2 (see legend and text).

increased OEF, has been reported [28, 38, 41]. This capacity of the brain to extract more oxygen to counterbalance the effects of a decrease in perfusion is, moreover, not restricted to cerebral infarction; it has long been noted in carotid artery ligation and occlusion, as well as in global cerebral ischemia either caused by systemic arterial hypotention, intracranial hypertension or hypocapnia [12]. Before the advent of ^{15}O PET studies, however, it was not known to occur focally in the brain of man.

The time course of changes in both CBF and OEF within the infarct could be approached from this study of 68 instances, including 7 infarcts studied twice. Strikingly, the 'misery-perfusion syndrome' has never been observed in infarcts older than 14 days, and was present in all 3 cases studied within the first 3 days after onset. Conversely, the 'luxury-perfusion syndrome' has been observed only later than 4 days (although no infarct dating less than 30 h has been studied, and thus a short-lasting 'luxury-perfusion syndrome' may have been overlooked) and earlier than 60 days after onset. Focal hyperemia was seen only between the 5th and the 20th day after onset, whereas more acute infarcts were characterized by a profound decrease in CBF that may represent the 'no-reflow' phenomenon [4]. Such a course of events is represented in figures 2 and 3, respectively, representing CBF and OEF within the infarct relative to the unaffected side. They clearly demonstrate the tendency of CBF to increase between the 2nd and the 20th day while the OEF conversely decreases in a mirror fashion. After this date, CBF decreases again while OEF tends to return to normal, presumably indicating progressive removal of necrotic tissue from the infarcted area. An illustrative example is shown in figure 4.

No definitive statement concerning the prognostic correlates – and therefore the potential therapeutic importance – of these two types of flow-metabolism uncoupling observed in cerebral infarction can be made yet, but a number of guidelines appear as a result of our experience. Focal 'luxury-perfusion', when severe, seems to indicate an unfavorable tissue prognosis as shown from topographic correlations with follow-up CT scan in a large number of cases [13], and with postmortem study in 1 case. *Ackerman* et al. [1] in cerebral infarction and *Obrist* et al. [29] in brain trauma reached similar conclusions. However, surrounding areas of less severe 'luxury-perfusion' have been associated with tissue long-term integrity – as far as can be judged from CT evidence – in a few instructive cases. There are, therefore, indications that 'luxury-perfusion' is indeed but a syndrome that may take place in irreversibly infarcted tissue as well as in surrounding tissue that may nevertheless spontaneously survive. Focal 'misery-perfusion', on the other hand, seems often predictive of potential tissue recovery: in one case of cerebral infarction (migrainous in nature), the area which showed 'misery-perfusion' seemed structurally intact as judged from clinical and CT data [14]. Spontaneous clinical regression in one of our patients with 'misery-perfusion' was spectacular, as in a similar case reported by *Ackerman* et al. [1]. Morever, in addition to cerebral infarction per se, we have observed focal 'misery-perfusion' in several cases in transient ischemic attacks (TIAs) distal to internal carotid artery (ICA) occlusion, including 1 patient with normal CT scan (fig. 5) and 2 other patients where CBF and OEF returned to normal following STA-MCA arterial bypass [11]. On the whole, therefore, 'misery-perfusion' may suggest that, although in a precarious state, the tissue in which it is located is potentially viable. However, in 2 patients with acute infarction, areas of brain tissue exhibiting the 'misery-perfusion syndrome', concomitant with almost zero focal blood flow, spontaneously underwent necrosis, as evidenced by CT scan in 1 case and postmortem in the other. Obviously, absolute quantitation of CBF, OEF and $CMRO_2$ may, in the near future, help define, within the above patterns of either luxury- or misery-perfusion syndromes, specific thresholds more accurately indicative of tissue viability. Hopefully, from such data, therapeutic implications will then be derived and the circulatory and metabolic responses to any therapeutic intervention will then be locally objectivized.

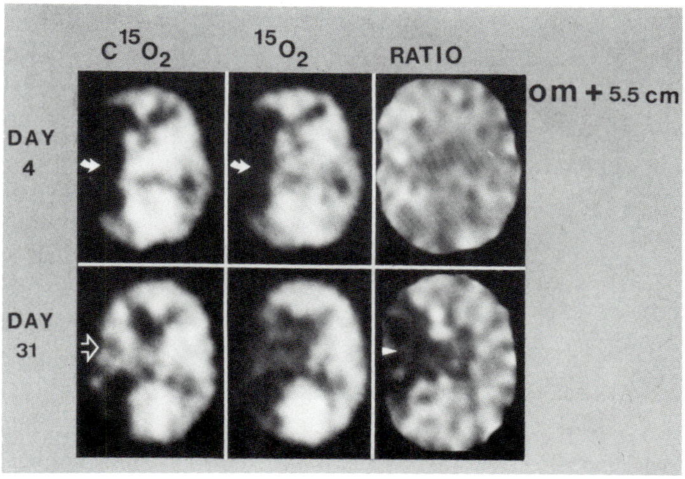

Fig. 4. Left MCA territory infarction studied at day 4 and day 31 after clinical onset. The tomographic images were taken at the 5.5 cm level above and roughly parallel to the orbitomeatal (OM) line. Left side is on the left (viewed from above). At day 4, there is a severe decrease in both $C^{15}O_2$ and $^{15}O_2$ count rate within the infarct (curved arrows) with a normal or slighly increased ratio value. At day 31, perfusion has returned in the infarct as evidenced by augmented $C^{15}O_2$ count rate (arrow frame), but the OEF is now profoundly decreased within the infarct (arrowhead) indicating the 'luxury-perfusion syndrome'.

The above clearly indicates the failure of conventional techniques which allow measurement of CBF only, using xenon-133 for example. An additional illustration of this point involves the problem of focal hyperemia in recent hemispheric infarction, classically considered as the formal indication of underlying 'luxury-perfusion': of the nine examples of focal hyperemia which we have observed, it was associated 5 times with decreased OEF, i.e. 'luxury-perfusion', but in the other 4 cases OEF was normal, implying post- or peri-ischemic hypermetabolism [20] with probably quite different prognostic meaning. *Yamaguchi* et al. [43] stressed the fact that tissue showing hyperemia after experimental arterial occlusion could still be structurally normal at subsequent pathological examination.

We shall say little about the results we have obtained in older hemispheric infarction (more than 6 weeks) which appears simply as a 'perfusion vacuum', a zone of zero blood flow, the contours of which can be exactly superimposed on the loss of substance observed on the CT scan [8]. More interesting is the fact that adjacent cerebral tissue seems to have, as far as can be assessed, close to normal perfusion and OEF.

Another crucial feature of cerebral infarction, now open to study by PET imaging, is the occurrence of functional depression remote from the site of injury, including the diaschisis phenomenon. A better understanding of the clinical correlates in completed stroke, as well as of the processes of the long-term partial clinical recovery, may now be at hand. Thus, metabolic depression of the cortical mantle and/or the thalamus ipsilateral to circumscribed superficial infarct have been observed in PET studies using ^{18}F-2-deoxy-glucose [25] as well as in our ^{15}O inhalation studies. The classical although controversial phenomenon of metabolic depression over the cerebral hemisphere contralateral to the infarct, thought to be secondary to 'transneural' deactivation [24], has received some support from PET studies [25]. In this respect, we have recently, for the first time, demonstrated that supratentorial infarction often induces a transitory metabolic de-

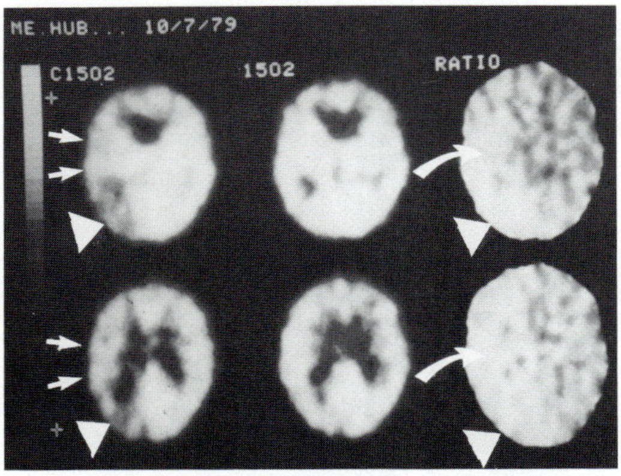

Fig. 5. Tomographic images taken at the OM + 5 cm (upper row) and OM + 7 cm (lower row) in a patient with left hemisphere TIAs and ipsilateral ICA occlusion. The patient was neurologically normal at the time of study. There is a decreased CBF over the left hemisphere (straight arrows), associated with an increased OEF (curved arrows), i.e., the 'misery perfusion syndrome'. Note that the abnormalities predominate at the parieto-occipital watershed areas (arrowheads).

pression in the contralateral cerebellar hemisphere [10]. This phenomenon, called 'crossed cerebellar diaschisis', suggests a transneural deactivation of the cerebrocerebellar loop, and may represent the early metabolic correlate of the crossed cerebellar atrophy sometimes observed in long-standing unilateral brain damage.

Still another point that has been identified by our studies concerns the problem of protracted hemodynamic failure distal to ICA occlusion [11]. The 4 patients studied were not stable following ICA occlusion (with the clinical picture of permanent – but sometimes progressive – deficit undergoing episodes of transient worsening) and usually showed CT evidence of circumscribed ipsilateral watershed infarctions at the MCA borderzones. The pathophysiologic correlate of this clinical situation was that of a decreased CBF with either normal or increased (i.e. 'misery-perfusion syndrome') OEF clearly predominating at the above-mentioned watershed territories, and far more extended than the CT abnormalities. Furthermore, since both CBF and OEF returned to normal following STA-MCA anastomosis, there is evidence that such changes are potentially reversible and are presumably indicative of impending extension of the watershed necrosis. In this category of patients, such patterns of watershed CBF-OEF abnormalities may thus constitute rational indications for STA-MCA bypass surgery. They also shed some light on the pathophysiological mechanisms of watershed infarction.

In summary, although only semiquantitative, the above results clearly indicate the usefulness of the ^{15}O continuous inhalation technique as a clinical research tool in the investigation of the pathophysiology of cerebral ischemic disorders. With the advent of both absolute quantitation of CBF and $CMRO_2$ and new PET devices of improved spatial resolution, this technique should gain a tremendous importance in neurological research.

Acknowledgements

Our warm thanks are given to *N. Duquesnoy, J. Sastre, M. Crouzel, C. Loc'h, C. Crouzel, P. Collard* and the cyclotron staff for their invaluable assistance.

References

1 Ackerman, R.H.; Alpert, N.M.; Correia, J.A.; Grotta, J.C.; Fallick, J.T.; Chang, J.Y.; Brownell, G.L.; Taveras, J.M.: Correlations of positron emission scans with TCT scans and clinical course. Acta neurol. scand. *60:* suppl. 72, pp. 230–231 (1979).

2 Ackerman, R.H.; Subramanyam, R.; Correia, J.; Alpert, N.A.; Taveras, J.M.: Positron imaging of cerebral blood flow during continuous inhalation of $C^{15}O_2$. Stroke *11:* 45–49 (1980).

3 Alpert, N.M.; Ackerman, R.H.; Correia, J.A.; Grotta, J.L.; Chang, J.Y.; Taveras, J.M.: Measurement of cerebral blood flow and oxygen metabolism in transverse section. Preliminary results. Acta neurol. scand. *60:* suppl. 72, pp. 196–197 (1979).

4 Ames, A., III; Wright, R.L.; Kowada, M.; et al.: Cerebral ischemia. II. The no-reflow phenomenon. Am. J. Path. *52:* 437–453 (1968).

5 Baron, J.C.; Comar, D.; Bousser, M.G.; Soussaline, F.; Crouzel, C.; Plummer, D.; Kellershohn, C.; Castaigne, P.: Etude tomographique chez l'homme, du débit sanguin et de la consommation d'oxygène du cerveau par inhalation continue d'oxygène 15. Revue neurol. *134:* 545–556 (1978).

6 Baron, J.C.; Comar, D.; Soussaline, F.; Todd-Pokopek, A.; Bousser, M.G.; Castaigne, P.; Kellershohn, C.: Continuous ^{15}O inhalation technique. An attempt to quantify CBF, EO_2 and $CMRO_2$. Acta neurol. scand. *60:* suppl. 72, pp. 194–195 (1979).

7 Baron, J.C.; Comar, D.; Bousser, M.G.; Plummer, D.; Loc'h, C.; Kellershohn, C.; Castaigne, P.: Patterns of CBF and oxygen extraction fraction (EO_2) in hemispheric infarcts. A tomography study with the ^{15}O inhalation technique. Acta neurol. scand. *60:* suppl. 72, pp. 324–325 (1979).

8 Baron, J.C.; Bousser, M.G.; Comar, D.; Kellershohn, C.: Human hemispheric infarction studied by positron emission tomography and the ^{15}O continuous inhalation technique; in Caille, Salamon, Computerized tomography, pp. 231–237 (Springer, Berlin 1980).

9 Baron, J.C.; Naquet, R.; Steinling, M.; Loc'h, C.; Soussaline, F.: Tomographic measurement of cerebral blood flow with the $C^{15}O_2$ continuous inhalation technique. Experimental evidence. Ann. Neurol. *8:* 99–100 (1980).

10 Baron, J.C.; Bousser, M.G.; Comar, D.; Castaigne, P.: 'Crossed cerebellar diaschisis' in human supratentorial infarction. Ann. Neurol. *8:* 128 (1980).

11 Baron, J.C.; Rey, A.; Guillard, A.; Bousser, M.G.; Comar, D.; Castaigne, P.: Non-invasive tomographic imaging of cerebral blood flow and oxygen extraction fraction in superficial temporal artery to middle cerebral artery anastomosis; in Proc. 10th Salzburg Conf. Cerebral Vascular Diseases. (Excerpta Medica, Amsterdam, in press).

12 Bes, A.; Geraud, G.: Circulation cérébrale (Physiopathologie, Sandoz, Paris 1974).

13 Blas, C.; Baron, J.C.; Iba-Zizen, M.T.; Bousser, M.G.; Cabanis, E.A.; Comar, D.; Bories, J.; Castaigne, P.: 9th Congr. Eur. Soc. Neuroradiology, Brussels 1980.

14 Bousser, M.G.; Baron, J.C.; Iba-Zizen, M.T.; Comar, D.; Cabanis, E.; Castaigne, P.: Migrainous cerebral infarction. A tomographic study of cerebral blood flow and oxygen extraction fraction with the oxygen 15 inhalation technique. Stroke *11:* 145–148 (1980).

15 Eichling, J.O.; Raichle, M.E.; Grubb, R.L.; Ter-Pogossian, M.M.: Evidence of the limitations of water as a freely diffusible tracer in brain of the rhesus monkey. Circulation Res. *35:* 358–364 (1974).

16 Fieschi, C.; Rosiers, M. des: Cerebral blood flow measurements in stroke; in Russel, Cerebral arterial disease pp. 85–106 (Pitman, Edinburgh 1976).

17 Frackowiak, R.S.J.; Lenzy, G.L.; Jones, T.; Heather, J.D.: Quantitative measurement of cerebral blood flow and oxygen metabolism in man using ^{15}O and positron emission tomography. Theory, procedure and normal values. J. Comput. Assist. Tomogr. (in press).

18 Ginsberg, M.D.; Reivich, M.: Use of the 2-deoxyglucose method of local cerebral glucose utilisation in the abnormal brain. Evaluation of the lumped constant during ischemia. Acta neurol. scand. *60:* suppl. 77, pp. 226–227 (1979).

19 Hoffman, E.J.; Huang, S.C.; Phelps, M.E.: Quantitation in positron emission computed tomography. I. Effect on object size. J. Comput. Assist Tomogr. *3:* 299–308 (1979).

20 Hossmann, K.A.; Sakaki, S.; Kimoto, K.: Cerebral uptake of glucose and oxygen in the cat brain after prolonged ischemia. Stroke *7:* 301–305 (1976).

21 Huang, S.C.; Phelps, M.E.; Hoffman, E.J.; Kuhl, D.E.: A theoretical study of quantitative flow measurements with constant infusion of short-lived isotopes. Physiol. med. Biol. *24:* 1151–1161 (1979).

22 Huang, S.C.; Hoffman, E.J.; Phelps, M.E.; Kuhl, D.E.: Quantitation in positron emission computed tomography. II. Effects of inaccurate attenuation

correction. J. Comput. assist. Tomogr. *3:* 804–814 (1979).

23 Jones, T.; Chesler, D.A.; Ter Pogossian, M.M.: The continuous inhalation of oxygen 15 for assessing regional oxygen extraction in the brain of man. Br. J. Radiol. *49:* 339–343 (1976).

24 Kempisky, W.H.: Experimental study of distant effects of acute focal injury. A study of diaschisis. Acta neurol. psychiat. *79:* 376–389 (1958).

25 Kuhl, D.E.; Phelps, M.E.; Kowell, A.P.; Metter, E.J.; Selin, C.; Winter, J.: Effects of stroke on local cerebral metabolism and perfusion. Mapping by emission computed tomography of ^{18}F-DG and $^{13}NH_3$. Ann. Neurol. *8:* 47–60 (1980).

26 Lassen, N.A.: The luxury-perfusion syndrome and its possible relation to acute metabolic acidosis localised within the brain. Lancet *ii:* 1113–1115 (1966).

27 Lenzi, G.L.; Jones, T.; McKenzie, C.G.; Buckingham, P.O.; Clark, J.C.; Moss, S.: Study of the regional cerebral metabolism and blood flow relationships in man using the method of continuously inhaling oxygen 15 and oxygen 15 labeled carbon dioxide. J. Neurol. Neurosurg. Psychiat. *41:* 1–10 (1978).

28 Meyer, J.S.: Circulatory changes following occlusion of the middle cerebral artery and their relation to function. J. Neurosurg. *15:* 653–673 (1958).

29 Obrist, W.D.; Genn-Arelli, T.A.; Segaka, H.; Dolinskas, C.A.; Langfitt, T.W.: Relation of cerebral blood flow to neurological status and outcome in head-injured patients. J. Neurosurg. *51:* 292–300 (1979).

30 Phelps, M.E.; Hoffman, E.J.; Raybaud, C.: Factors which affect cerebral uptake and retention of $^{13}NH_3$. Stroke *8:* 694–701 (1977).

31 Phelps, M.E.; Hoffman, E.J.; Huang, S.C.; Kuhl, D.E.; et al.. A new computerized tomographic imaging system for positron-emitting radiopharmaceuticals. J. nucl. Med. *19:* 636–647 (1978).

32 Phelps, M.E.; Huang, S.C.; Hoffman, E.J., et al.: Tomographic measurement of local cerebral glucose metabolic rate in humans with (F-18)2-fluoro-2-deoxy-*D*-glucose. Validation of method. Ann. Neurol. *6:* 371–388 (1979).

33 Raichle, M.E.: Quantitative in vivo autoradiography with positron emission tomography. Brain Res. Rev. *1:* 47–68 (1979).

34 Raichle, M.E.; Welch, M.J.; Grubb, R.L.; Larson, K.B.; Laux, B.E.; Ter Pogossian, M.M.: Regional cerebral oxygen utilization with positron emission tomography. Ann. Neurol. *7:* 157 (1979).

35 Reivich, M.; Kuhl, D.; Wolf, A.; et al.: The ^{18}F fluorodeoxyglucose method for the measurement of local cerebral glucose utilization in man. Circulation Res. *44:* 127–137 (1979).

36 Soussaline, F.; Todd-Prokopek, A.E.; Plummer, D.; Comar, D.; Loc'h, C.; Houle, S.; Kellershohn, C.: The physical performances of a single slice positron tomographic system and preliminary results in a clinical environment. Eur. J. nucl. Med. *4:* 237–249 (1979).

37 Subramanyam, R.; Alpert, N.M.; Hoop, B.; Brownell, G.L.; Taveras, J.M.: A model for regional cerebral oxygen distribution during continuous inhalation of $^{15}O_2$, $C^{15}O$ and $C^{15}O_2$. J. nucl. Med. *19:* 48–53 (1978).

38 Symon, L.; Ross Russel, R.W.: The development of cerebral collateral circulation following occlusion of vessels in the neck. J. neurol. Sci. *13:* 197–208 (1971).

39 Ter-Pogossian, M.M.; Phelps, M.E.; Hoffman, E.J.; Mullani, N.A.: A positron-emission transaxial tomograph for nuclear imaging (PETT). Radiology *114:* 89–98 (1975).

40 Thomas, D.J.; Jones, T.: The combined use of the intravenous xenon-133 technique and the $^{15}O_2$ inhalation method; in Greenhalgh, Rose, Progress in stroke research, vol. I, pp. 330–339 (Pitman Medical, Bath 1979).

41 Waltz, A.G.; Sundt, T.M.: The microvasculature and microcirculation of the cerebral cortex after arterial occlusion. Brain *90:* 681–696 (1967).

42 Waltz, A.G.: Red venous blood. Occurrence and significance in ischemic and non-ischemic cerebral cortex. J. Neurosurg. *31:* 141–147 (1969).

43 Yamaguchi, T.; Waltz, A.G.; Okazaki, H.: Hyperemia and ischemia in experimental cerebral infarction. Correlation of histo-pathology and regional blood flow. Neurology, Minneap. *21:* 565–578 (1971).

44 Yamamoto, Y.L.; Thomson, C.J.; Meyer, E.; Robertson, J.S.; Feindel, W.: Dynamic positron emission tomography for study of cerebral remodynamics in a cross-section of the head using positron-emitting 68 Ga-EDTA and 77 Kr. J. Comput. Assist. Tomogr. *1:* 43–56 (1977).

J.C. Baron, Service Hospitalier Frédéric-Joliot, Hôpital d'Orsay, F–91406 Orsay (France)

Eur. Neurol. *20:* 285–290 (1981)

$CMRO_2$ and CBF by the Oxygen-15 Inhalation Technique

Results in Normal Volunteers and Cerebrovascular Patients

G.L. Lenzi[a], *R.S.J. Frackowiak*[b], *T. Jones*[b], *J.D. Heather*[b], *A.A. Lammertsma*[b], *C.G. Rhodes*[b], *C. Pozzilli*[a,1]

[a] Department of Neurology, IIIa Cattedra, University of Rome, Italy; [b] Medical Research Council, Cyclotron Unit, and Department of Medicine RPMS, Hammersmith Hospital, London, England

Key Words. Cerebral blood flow · Cerebral metabolism · Positron emission tomography · Cerebrovascular disorders

Abstract. The oxygen-15 inhalation technique has been applied to the quantitation of regional CBF, $CMRO_2$ and OER with positron emission tomography. The introduction of corrections for gamma-ray attenuation, and for recirculation, has allowed us to obtain values for CBF, $CMRO_2$ and OER in close agreement with values obtained using other techniques. In 27 normal volunteers mean $CMRO_2$ shows values ranging from 4.98 to 3.79 ml/100 ml/min, depending on the region evaluated. Mean CBF values range from 55.3 to 38.8 ml/100 ml/min. Mean OER is more constant, ranging from 0.56 to 0.49, with a mean of 0.53 ± 0.04, thus reflecting the close matching between metabolism and blood supply. We have further identified corrections for cerebral blood volume, which is measurable, and for water partition coefficient, which remains uncertain. In preliminary studies these corrections decrease the OER over the physiological range of flow by 10%, with a 15% lower $CMRO_2$. The reproducibility of the results and the effects of aging have been studied. A series of 27 studies on acute ischaemic CVD are reported. The course of the clinical condition has been correlated with the quantitation of oxygen utilization and blood flow performed at different intervals from the onset of symptoms.

Introduction

The development of positron emission tomographic (PET) techniques now allows the study of cerebral metabolism and blood flow in men, non-invasively and at a regional level.

The two major substrates of cerebral metabolism, glucose and oxygen, have been recently labeled with positron emitters and utilized in normal volunteers and in several neurological conditions [see *Lenzi* et al., in press].

1 Dr. *A.A. Lammertsma* is a fellow of 'Stichting Koningin Wilhelmina Fonds', The Dutch Society for Cancer Research. Dr. *G.L. Lenzi* was partly supported by CNR grants No. 78.02653.04 and 79.02161.04. Dr. *R.S.J. Frackowiak* is in receipt of a MRC Training Fellowship.

Table I. Mean values for rCBF, $rCMRO_2$ and rOER for grey (G) and white (W) matter in normal volunteers (column A), also divided in two subgroups, below 50 years (column B) and above 50 years (column C)

		A (n = 27)	B: 'young' group < 50 years (n = 16)	C: 'old' group > 50 years (n = 11)
CBF	G	64.5 ± 17.33	72.63 ± 20.88	52.68 ± 12.17
	W	21.16 ± 2.74	21.21 ± 2.81	21.09 ± 2.65
$CMRO_2$	G	5.74 ± 1.12	6.5 ± 1.47	4.64 ± 0.60
	W	1.84 ± 0.34	1.90 ± 0.44	1.75 ± 0.20
OER	G	0.49 ± 0.10	0.48 ± 0.10	0.50 ± 0.11
	W	0.47 ± 0.09	0.47 ± 0.10	0.47 ± 0.08

The purpose of this paper is to summarize the results obtained at the Hammersmith Hospital, after 1 year of experience.

Therory, Methods and Materials

The oxygen-15 inhalation technique was first applied clinically by our group in 1977 [*Lenzi* et al., 1977, 1978a,b] using non-tomographic measurements.

The technique consists of two repeated procedures: in the first the patient breathes oxygen-15 labeled carbon dioxide ($C^{15}O_2$) at physiological concentrations; in the second, labeled molecular oxygen ($^{15}O_2$) is inhaled.

The first procedure allows the quantitation of rCBF if the concentration of the isotope ($H_2{}^{15}O$) in the arterial blood and cerebral tissues is known.

The second procedure results in a total equilibrium activity in the brain due to the sum of the three components: metabolically produced labeled water, recirculating labeled water and the ^{15}O-labeled molecular oxygen attached to haemoglobin in the vascular compartment.

Dividing the cerebral activity obtained during $^{15}O_2$ inhalation by that obtained during $C^{15}O_2$ inhalation, and correcting for recirculating water by appropriate measurements, the oxygen extraction ratio (rOER) is obtained [see *Frackowiak* et al., in press].

Finally one obtains the cerebral metabolic rate for oxygen ($rCMRO_2$) from the relationship:

$rCMRO_2$ = rCBF × rOER × total blood oxygen content.

It follows that the distribution of ^{15}O during continuous $^{15}O_2$ inhalation does not reliably represent cerebral oxygen metabolism.

Two major corrections have been identified in the method: (1) an absolute correction for attenuation, which is measured with a 'transmission' scan at the same cerebral levels as the metabolic and circulatory studies, and (2) a correction for the blood volume component.

This second correction was not routinely performed in the studies here reported. Therefore, the values for $CMRO_2$ and OER are overestimated by 15% and 10%, respectively, while CBF is not significantly affected by this factor.

27 studies on normal volunteers and 27 on patients presenting with ischemic cerebrovascular disease have been performed. 10 normal volunteers have been studied twice at different intervals ranging from 1 h to 10 months.

In CVD patients, the first study was performed as soon as possible after the onset of symptoms; subsequent follow ups were repeated at weekly intervals.

Results

Normal Studies

Table I shows the mean values for rCBF, $rCMRO_2$ and rOER for grey and white matter (insula and centrum semiovale respectively)

Table II. Mean regional values for CBF, $CMRO_2$ and OER in 27 normal men (each value represents the mean value in a region of volume 1.6 cm × 5 cm^2)

	Occipital	Visual	Parietal	Motor	Frontal	Insula
Left hemisphere						
rCBF	44.8	44.9	38.8	45.5	46.5	54.5
$rCMRO_2$	4.58	4.44	3.79	4.29	4.32	4.88
rOER	0.55	0.52	0.53	0.51	0.50	0.49
Right hemisphere						
rCBF	47.0	47.6	40.4	49.3	43.6	55.3
$rCMRO_2$	4.83	4.71	3.90	4.66	4.01	4.98
rOER	0.56	0.53	0.52	0.51	0.50	0.49

Table III. Mean regional values for CBF, $CMRO_2$ and OER in 11 normal volunteers older than 50 years (same sampling as in table II)

	Occipital	Visual	Parietal	Motor	Frontal	Insula
rCBF	39.7	40.2	38.8	40.1	41.0	45.7
OER	0.57	0.54	0.53	0.53	0.51	0.50
$CMRO_2$	4.01	3.83	3.65	3.80	3.80	3.96

in our series of 27 observations on normal volunteers (column A). Dividing our normal population in two groups, the 'young' group, with subjects below 50 years of age, and the 'old' group, with subjects above 50 years of age, we have obtained the relative values for rCBF, $rCMRO_2$ and rOER in these two groups (columns B and C).

Table II shows the mean values for rCBF, $rCMRO_2$ and rOER for the grey matter in 12 cerebral regions of volume 1.6 cm × 5 cm^2. These differ from the former by representing heterogeneous mixtures of the appropriate cortex and underlying white matter. The values quoted therefore strictly represent mean weighted indexes of rCBF, $rCMRO_2$ and rOER and are also subject to the partial volume effect [*Hoffman* et al., 1979]. The 12 windows have been selected for the OM + 4 cm plane and correspond to the anatomical regions indicated in the table. We have choosen this fairly rigid form of data analysis in order to avoid subjectivity in defining the regions of interest on the scans.

Reproducibility

The reproducibility of results was tested in two 'acute' (30–60 min) and 8 long-term (1–10 months) experiments. In the 'acute' reproducibility studies, $rCMRO_2$ and rCBF vary from 4 to 10%, depending on the region evaluated. We are actually expanding the number of these studies in order to obtain a reliable statistic of the 'acute' reproducibility. In 8

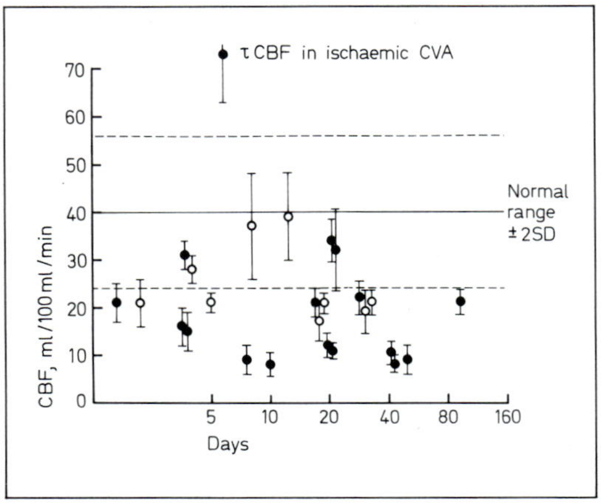

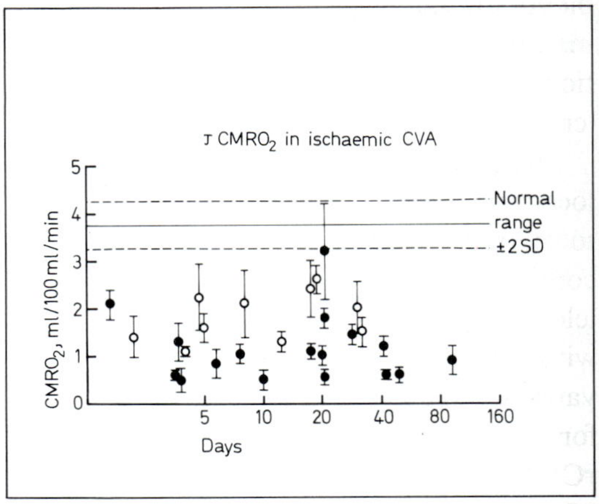

1

Fig. 1. rCBF in the ischaemic CVA: mean value of a region of volume = 1.6 cm × 5 cm², representing the core of the lesion. ○ = Patients with subsequent clinical improvement; ● = patients with stationary or worsening clinical outcome. In the graph the level 40 ± 16 ml/100 ml/min represents the mean CBF in the 'old' group of normal volunteers, ± 2 SD of the regional variability.

Fig. 2. rCMRO$_2$ in the ischaemic CVA: same sampling from the same region as in the figure 1. ○ = Improved; ● = stationary or worse.

'long-term' reproducibility tests, mean CMRO$_2$ varied by ± 10%, mean CBF by ± 16%. At the regional level, some cerebral regions, such as the motor and the calcarine cortices, were more stable (rCMRO$_2$ variability ± 4.7%; rCBF variability ± 14.6%), while frontal and associative visual cortices showed a markedly larger variability (rCMRO$_2$ 15.8%; rCBF = 19%).

Aging

Aging affects both rCMRO$_2$ and rOER. In normal volunteers older than 50 years, a mean decrease of 30% was observed in CMRO$_2$ and CBF, when compared with the younger group (table I). OER remains stable in old age, thus once again reflecting the coupling between flow and metabolism.

The decrease in CBF and CMRO$_2$ is more evident for regions such as the visual cortex and the insula, probably reflecting the loss of neurons from these regions where the relative amount of 'grey' matter is greater in the sampled volume (see 'Discussion').

Table III shows the values for rCBF, rCMRO$_2$ and rOER in 11 normal volunteers over 50 years old.

Cerebrovascular Diseases

A series of 27 studies on CVD patients has been performed. 9 studies have been performed during the first 7 days after the onset of clinical signs and symptoms, 11 after 7 and before 22 days, and 7 after 22 and before 90 days. All patients presented clinically with acute stroke. The study has been repeated twice in 5 patients and three times in 4 patients.

Figures 1 and 2 show the behaviour of rCMRO$_2$ and rCBF in the ischaemic lesion. From the figures it appears that in general the oxygen metabolism is more affected than the blood flow 'in' the lesion. There is in the large majority a 'relative luxury perfusion' situation, while 'absolute luxury perfusion' and 'critical perfusion' are definitely rarer.

In addition, constant 'remote' effects of a localized lesion have been observed, referred to as 'transneuronal diaschisis'. These effects consist of a metabolic depression not paralleled by any similar decrease in CBF. Notwithstanding the small amount of observations, it appears that there are thresholds for no-recovery: 1–1.5 ml/100 ml/min for $rCMRO_2$ and 15–20 ml/100 ml/min for rCBF. However, an rCBF above 20 ml/100 ml/min does not necessarily correlate with an improvement in the clinical condition, though 9 of the 10 cases which had a good final outcome had a $rCMRO_2$ superior to 1.5 ml/100 ml/min. Of the 17 studies in patients with a poor outcome, 5 had a $CMRO_2$ above this threshold, though in 2 the final outcome could be considered independent of the cerebral lesion.

Discussion

The oxygen-15 inhalation technique and its utilization with PET has been discussed in detail in separate papers and we refer to these publications [*Frackowiak* et al., in press; *Lenzi* et al., 1980].

We will devote a brief discussion to three major points, namely: (1) the 'landscape' of the brain; (2) the effects of aging, and (3) the effects of ischaemic CVD.

The Cerebral 'Landscape'

A resting landscape of regional cerebral blood flow has been described by *Ingvar and Lassen* [1975] using the intracarotid Xe-133 technique.

We have analysed our data regionally using the windowing technique of twelve regions described above. The regional variation of CBF and $CMRO_2$ are shown in table II. It has to be underlined that *our* values were obtained on a 'steady-state' condition, by recording the activity for 5 min, while the intracarotid approach records the wash-out curve for the first 1 or 2 min after the injection. This difference may lead to a more homogeneous landscape in *our* studies.

A striking difference between this and the intracarotid landscape is the lack of hyperfrontal pattern [*Ingvar,* 1975]. This difference may be due to the non-invasiveness of the oxygen-15 inhalation technique compared to the intracarotid approach. Anxiety, pain and mentation, are thought to activate the frontal regions in particular. The greater stimulation of the intracarotid method is to be compared with the relaxed, often drowsy, subject who is inhaling isotope.

The Effects of Aging

Previous results on the effect of aging on CBF and $CMRO_2$ [*Kety,* 1956; *Scheinberg* et al., 1953] have been confirmed. In general the decrease in mean $CMRO_2$ parallels that of mean CBF.

The fall off in metabolism cannot be due to a primary flow decrease, because the mean OER remains stable throughout aging.

If the fall off in oxygen utilization were secondary to a primary subclinical ischaemia, a rise in OER would be expected. In other words, aging does not mean 'critical perfusion'.

The Effects of Ischaemic CVD

We must underline that the number of cases studied so far is too limited to draw general conclusions. Therefore, we prefer to summarize the main observations in four statements: (1) there is no constant pattern of rCBF, $rCMRO_2$ and rOER changes in ischaemic CVD; (2) $rCMRO_2$ correlates with clinical conditions and final outcome; (3) wide-spread and 'remote' effects of a localized lesion are constantly observed, and (4) a very large number of patients will have to be studied in the immediate period after the acute event with repeated follow-up, before final indications for therapy can be drawn in a rigorous scientific manner.

References

Frackowiak, R.S.J.; Lenzi, G.L.; Jones, T.; Heather, J.D.: The quantitative measurement of regional cerebral blood flow and oxygen metabolism in man using oxygen-15 and positron emission tomography: theory, procedure and normal values. J. Comput. assist. Tomogr. (in press).

Hoffman, E.J.; Huang, S.C.; Phelps, M.E.: Quantitation in positron emission computed tomography. I. Effect of object size. J. Comput. assist. Tomogr. *3:* 299–308 (1979).

Ingvar, D.H.: Patterns of brain activity revealed by measurements of regional cerebral blood flow; in Brain work. A. Beyzon Symp. VIII, pp. 397–413 (Munksgaard, Copenhagen 1975).

Ingvar, D.H.; Lassen, N.A.: Regulation of cerebral blood flow; in Himwich, Brain metabolism and cerebral disorders, 2nd ed., pp. 181–206 (Spectrum Publications, New York 1975).

Lenzi, G.L.; Jones, T.; McKenzie, C.G.; Buckingham, L.D.; Clark, J.C.; Moss, S.: A study of regional cerebral metabolism and blood flow relationships in man using the method of continuously inhaling oxygen-15 and oxygen-15 labelled carbon dioxide. J. Neurol. Neurosurg. Psychiat. *41:* 1–10 (1978a).

Lenzi, G.L.; Jones, T.; McKenzie, C.G.; Moss, S.: Regional studies of oxygen uptake and blood flow in chronic cerebrovascular disorders using the oxygen inhalation technique; in Meyer, Lechner, Reivich, Cerebral vascular disease, pp. 187–190 (Excerpta Medica, Amsterdam 1977).

Lenzi, G.L.; Jones, T.; McKenzie, C.G.; Moss, S.: A non-invasive regional study of chronic cerebrovascular disorders using the oxygen-15 inhalation technique (OIT). J. Neurol. Neurosurg. Psychiat. *41:* 11–17 (1978b).

Lenzi, G.L.; Jones, T.; Frackowiak, R.S.J.: Positron emission tomography: state of the art in neurology. Adv. nucl. Med. (in press).

Kety, S.S.: Human cerebral blood flow and oxygen consumption as related to ageing. Ass. Res. nerv. Dis. Proc. *35:* 31–45 (1956).

Scheinberg, P.,; Blackburn, I.; Rich, M.; Saslaw, M.: Effects of aging on cerebral circulation and metabolism. AMA Archs Neurol. Psychiat. *70:* 77–85 (1953)

Dr. G.L. Lenzi, Department of Neurology,
IIIa Cattedra, University of Rome, Rome (Italy)

Eur. Neurol. *20:* 291–293 (1981)

Regional Activation of Brain Cortex in Man Revealed by ^{133}Xe Inhalation Flow Tomography

(with 1 color plate)

Niels A. Lassen

Department of Clinical Physiology, Bispebjerg Hospital, Copenhagen, Denmark

Local increases in cortex blood flow associated with increased neuronal function and metabolism of that same local area have been amply documented. The pattern of changes varies with the task performed in a highly meaningful manner. In man the most detailed maps have been obtained by the intraarterial ^{133}Xe injection method [1]. It involves the potential trauma inherent in the injection and only shows a part of one hemisphere in two dimensions (thus, superposition of tissue layers cannot be avoided).

Emission tomography of cerebral blood flow or metabolism is atraumatic and yields three-dimensional information in form of a series of slices of brain tissue. Using positron (dual photon) emitters and fluor-18-deoxyglucose, preliminary results showing cortical activation in man have been published [2, 3]. This study concerns similar findings using single-photon emission tomography of inhaled ^{133}Xe by a highly sensitive fast-rotating tomograph [4]. ^{133}Xe flow tomograms of normal subjects studied at rest and during brain activity show the active areas as regions of preferential flow increase.

Methods

The single-photon tomograph (Tomomatic-64, Medimatic Inc., Copenhagen, Denmark) is termed 'dynamic' as its fast-speed rotation (180 °/5 s) allows one to collect all the projections needed for reconstruction in so short an interval that they can be considered simultaneous in relation to the fairly slow arrival and washout of ^{133}Xe. Thus, superimposing many rotations, to obtain a sufficient number of impulses for adequate reconstruction (0.3–1.0 $\times$ 10^6), a time-averaged mean concentration of ^{133}Xe in each pixel is obtained [4].

In order to secure high sensitivity, each one of the three slices of brain tissue looked at, despite only being 2 cm thick, is recorded by 4 cm of crystal length. The instrument has four banks of detectors each consisting of 16 crystals. With the fairly open collimator used that resolution (FWMH) is about 1.7 cm in the plane and, as just mentioned, about 2 cm in the z direction [4]. During 1 min of ^{133}Xe inhalation (10 mCi/l) and for 3 min after, a sequence of four 1-min ^{133}Xe tomograms are recorded from three slices of the brain.

At the same time the arterial ^{133}Xe concentration curve is estimated by a single nonmoving scintillation detector placed over the right lung. The ^{133}Xe flow maps are calculated from the four pictures using the arterial curve [5, 6]. A convolution procedure is used assuming each pixel to represent an essentially homogeneous area having a monoexponential pulse-response function. A fixed tissue: blood partition coefficient (λ) of 1.15 is employed.

The radiation dose per study is about 0.3 rad for the target organ (the lung) and tenfold less for the gonads [7].

Results

Resting State

In the relaxed awake state with closed eyes the normal-flow tomograms are symmetrical: the side-to-side differences do not exceed 5%. The lowest tomographic slice has its midslice plane 2 cm above the orbito-meatal plane (OM + 2 cm). At this level the highest flow of about 60–80 ml/100 g/min is seen in the peripheral areas, lower in the deep parts of the brain comprising basal ganglia and thalamus, no sharply defined structures can be discerned. The middle tomographic slice has its midslice plane 6 cm above the orbito-meatal plane (OM + 6 cm). It shows high flow in the midline anteriorly (mesial frontal cortex), in the midline posteriorly (striate cortex), and in both lateral regions (sylvian cortex). The uppermost slice (OM + 10 cm) is the smallest cutting in part tangentially through much cortical tissue; a rather uniform high flow map is typically obtained.

Hand Movement

Rythmical movements of one hand in form of fist clenching at a rate of approximately 1/s results in normal man in an *asymmetry* in the uppermost slice (OM + 10 cm). Here a flow increase of 10–15 ml/100 g/min (about 20 %) is seen in the contralateral hand region, namely about in the middle of the slice towards the surface (fig. 1).

Discussion

The tomographic sensorimotor hand area corresponds to known anatomical localization. No other areas were seen active. In particular, we could not discern the supplementary motor area in the mesial frontal cortex. More complex motor tests may be needed to activate it sufficiently to be seen.

Using the ^{133}Xe intraarterial injection method and a battery of stationary detectors, the hand movement test used gives rise to a flow increase of about 30–40%. The field of each detector is a truncated tissue cone traversing all layers of the injected hemisphere. Hence, a superposition of active and nonactive cortex layers cannot be avoided. Could one see the primary sensorimotor cortex alone, excluding other tissue layers, one would expect much higher flow increase. Preliminary studies with the deoxyglucose autoradiographic method in monkeys point to metabolic increase of 100% in the primary sensorimotor hand area during complex hand-arm movements [*Sokoloff,* personal commun.].

Our ^{133}Xe flow tomograms may be compared to the focal flow metabolism increases seen with the fluor-18-deoxyglucose in man. These preliminary studies point to effects in the order of only 10% [2, 3]. This modest response is about the same as ours and of only about one tenth of the supposed 'true' response could one have seen solely the active cortex. Poor spatial resolution, Compton scatter, and the 'partial volume effect', all must be taken into account to explain this difficulty. The partial volume effect is presumably the most important factor: it stems from the fact that each pixel, measuring about 1.5 × 1.5 × 2.0 cm in our case, contains many tissue components of grey as well

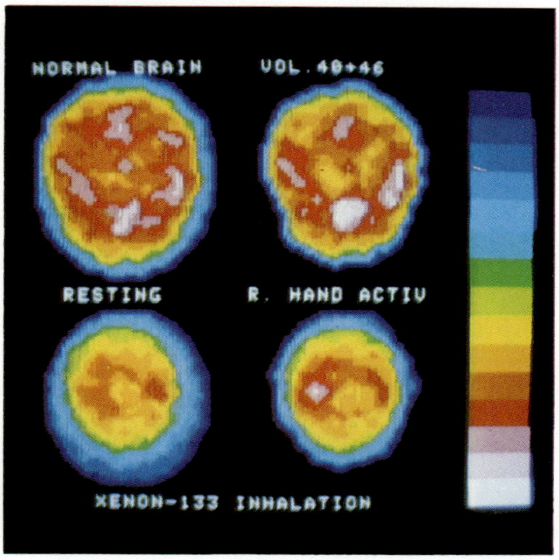

Fig. 1. Middle (OM + 6 cm) and upper (OM + 10 cm) slice in a normal subject at rest and during right-hand movement. The flow increase in the right motor cortex in upper slice is apparent.

as white matter. Hence, assuming homogeneity, as one does for calculating flow or metabolism, an appreciable error is committed. Using in each volume the measured average value, the high-flow components in part of the volume are deemphasized. Using ^{133}Xe inhalation, the uptake is, moreover, not quite linear with flow, the high-flow areas taking less than proportional to the flow relative to low-flow areas. Thus, the average concentration is not proportional to the average flow.

The partial volume effect here discussed does not influence the ^{133}Xe intraarterial method as it is used for disclosing the cortical activity. For this purpose the initial slope cortex blood flow calculation is used, a calculation much weighted in favor of the high-flow components. Had one instead used the height-over-area equation giving the average flow equally weighted for all flow levels, then the rapid early component would become submerged and the activation effects much attenuated (at least by a factor of three). If one as with the tomograph made a flow weighted for low flow, it is perhaps not surprising that an actual 100% effect, a doubling of flow, reduces to the level of 10–15%.

In conclusion, the tomographic mapping of brain function based on flow or metabolism seems at the present level of resolution reached to have insufficient resolution for effective mapping of active cortex in man. The resolution in the order of 1.5 cm^3 for both positron and single-photon emission tomography is inadequate. It seems, therefore, that the techniques are best suited for studying low flow/low metabolic states, a problem of major clinical importance. With improved instrument resolution the situation will be different.

References

1 Lassen, N.A.; Ingvar, D.H.; Skinhøj, E.: Brain function and blood flow. Scient. Am. *239:* 62–71 (1978).

2 Reivich, M.; Kuhl, D.; Wolf, A.; Greenberg, J.; Phelps, M.; Ido, T.; Casella, V.; Fowler, J.; Gallagher, B.; Hoffmann, E.; Alavi, A.; Sokoloff, L.: Measurement of local cerebral glucose metabolism in man with 18-F-2-fluoro-2-deoxy-*D*-glucose. Acta neur. scand. *56:* suppl. 64, pp. 190–191 (1977).

3 Kuhl, D.E.; Phelps, M.E.; Kowell, A.P.; Metter, E.J.; Selin, C.; Winter, J.: Effects of stroke on local cerebral metabolism and perfusion. Mapping by emission computed tomography of 18-FDG and 13-NH_3. Ann. Neurol. *8:* 47–60 (1980).

4 Stokely, E.M.; Sveinsdottir, E.; Lassen, N.A.; Rommer, P.: A single photon dynamic computer-assisted tomograph (DCAT) for imaging brain function in multiple cross-sections. J. Comput. assist. Tomogr. *4:* 230–240 (1980).

5 Kanno, I.; Lassen, N.A.: Two methods for calculating regional cerebral blood flow from emission computed tomography of inert gas concentrations. J. Comput. assist. Tomogr. *3:* 71–76 (1979).

6 Celsis, P.; Lassen, N.A.: (in preparation, 1980).

7 Atkins, H.L.; Robertson, J.S.; Croft, B.Y.; Tsui, B.; Susskind, H.; Ellis, K.J.; Loken, M.K.; Trevas, S.: Estimates of radiation absorbed doses from radioxenons in lung imaging. J. nucl. Med. *21:* 459–465 (1980).

Niels A. Lassen, MD, Department of Clinical Physiology, Bispebjerg Hospital,
DK–2400 Copenhagen NV (Denmark)

Eur. Neurol. *20:* 294–296 (1981)

Measurements of Regional Cerebral Blood Flow and Metabolism in Psychopathological States

David H. Ingvar[1]

Department of Clinical Neurophysiology, University Hospital, Lund, Sweden

Key Words. rCBF · Focal epilepsy · Organic dementia · Schizophrenia

Abstract. In different psychopathological states like focal epilepsy, organic dementia, and chronic schizophrenia, rCBF studies have previously demonstrated specific changes of the normal cerebral perfusion landscape. It has been assumed that these abnormalities – the hyperemia in epileptic foci, the regional reduction pattern in dementia as well as the abnormal flow distribution in chronic schizophrenia – represent metabolic alterations. Recent studies with positron emission tomography give solid support to this hypothesis. The glucose uptake in epileptic foci is increased and the uptake in the frontal cortex is reduced in chronic schizophrenia.

The metabolic studies show that regional cerebral activity in various psychopathological states is now accessible to a detailed study.

Introduction

This paper deals with some important regional cerebral circulatory abnormalities found in psychological states like in focal epilepsy, organic dementia and chronic schizophrenia. These abnormalities will then be related to some recent studies of the regional glucose uptake in the same disorders, measured with 18-fluoro-deoxyglucose and positron emission tomography.

[1] Supported by the Swedish Medical Research Council (No. B81-14X-00084-17C) and the Wallenberg Foundation.

Focal Epilepsy

Jackson's [14] well-known assumption that the epileptic focus contains masses of synchronously discharging nerve cells, has obtained much unequivocal support over the years. Electrophysiological studies with micro- and macrotechniques (EEG) have shown paroxysmal unit and mass discharges within the focal area [1]. Several studies with quantitative techniques have shown that such neuronal activity is accompanied by a focal hyperemia [13]. In human studies this was later confirmed by the quantitative ^{133}Xe clearance technique [7]. In some patients the rCBF method appeared superior to the EEG for localization of active foci, a fact which might be taken advantage of in neurosurgical therapy of focal epilepsy [6].

Recently, *Kuhl* et al. [15] have demonstrated the superiority of the three-dimensional positron emission tomography for the localization of epileptogenic foci. They used the 18-FDG method based upon the principle devised by *Sokoloff* [17]. The studies of *Kuhl* et al. [15] showed that the glucose utilization in an active epileptogenic focal area may amount to 3–4 times the normal mean for cerebral gray matter. Furthermore, a focal seizure 'drains' the surrounding cortex as well as the contralateral hemisphere which may show a subnormal metabolism. Finally, in the nonactive interictal phase, the focus may show a subnormal metabolism also, a finding confirming some observations with the rCBF technique [7]. This supports the notion of an epileptogenic region as a gray matter scar in which the vascular (capillary) bed is reduced and the neurons are injured and working at a subnormal level in the interictal phase – and at a supernormal level during the actual seizure.

Organic Dementia

In organic dementia, studies with quantitative methods like the nitrous oxide technique and the ^{133}Xe clearance technique, have shown that there is a reduction of the global (total mean) cerebral blood flow – and oxygen uptake – which is proportional to the intellectual deficit [5, 16]. To judge from recent studies, this general conclusion appears to hold for all types of organic dementia, be they degenerative (Alzheimer, Pick, Jacob Creutzfeldt), cerebrovascular, or posttraumatic [12] in origin.

Multiregional rCBF studies have furthermore demonstrated that there are important *regional* correlations [5]. Thus, memory deficits in organic dementia are accompanied by a low blood flow in the temporal regions. Symptoms of agnosia go with a low flow in parietooccipital regions. Speech difficulties may show various regional flow decreases depending upon whether the symptoms have mainly expressive or impressive character [4]. There is therefore evidence that the rCBF landscape in organic dementia conveys information on the localization of the subsymptoms pertaining to the general syndrome of dementia. Interestingly enough, the low flow areas also correspond fairly closely to those in which the loss of neurons is most pronounced [9].

So far, no regional cerebral metabolic studies of patients with organic dementia have been published in which positron emission tomography has been used. It might be predicted that such studies with sufficient spatial resolution may enhance our knowledge considerably about the localization and the severity of the cerebral metabolic and circulatory abnormalities which ultimately shape the symptomatology seen in individual patients suffering from organic dementia.

Chronic Schizophrenia

In a series of papers it has been shown that chronic schizophrenia is accompanied by an abnormal distribution of the cerebral blood flow [3, 8, 10, 11]. The normally high blood flow in frontal areas (at rest) is proportionally lower the most autism, inactivity and catatonic symptoms the patients showed. The flow occipito-parieto-temporally is high, the more so, the more cognitive disturbance the patients showed. There is reason to assume that this maldistribution – which does not affect the total mean cerebral blood flow (or oxygen uptake) may be caused by some defect(s) in projection systems to the cortex from the brain stem, possibly also involving the basal ganglia [8].

Recently, *Farkas* et al. [2] reported a series of positron emission tomography studies in chronic schizophrenics. They also found that such patients have a significantly lower glucose utilization in the frontal lobes. Thus, it appears to have been confirmed that the low flow frontally in chronic schizophrenia represents an abnormally low metabolism in this part of the brain. Emission tomography with higher resolution will undoubtedly clarify further details of the maldistribution of cerebral metabolism which apparently forms a basic part of the cerebral dysfunction in chronic schizophrenia.

References

1 Ajmone-Marsan, C.; Ralston, B.L.: The epileptic seizure (Thomas, Springfield 1957).
2 Farkas, et al.: Am. Soc. biol. Psychiat., Meet., Boston 1980.
3 Franzén, G.; Ingvar, D.H.: Abnormal distribution of cerebral activity in chronic schizophrenia. J. psychiat. Res. *12:* 199–214 (1975).
4 Gustafson, L.; Hagberg, B.; Ingvar, D.H.: Speech disturbances in presenile dementia related to local cerebral blood flow abnormalities in the dominant hemisphere. Brain Language *5:* 103–118 (1978).
5 Hagberg, B.; Ingvar, D.H.: Cognitive reduction in presenile dementia related to regional abnormalities of the cerebral blood flow. Br. J. Psychiat. *128:* 209–222 (1976).
6 Hougaard, K.; Oikawa, T.; Sveinsdottir, E.; Skinhöj, E.; Ingvar, D.H.; Lassen, N.A.: Regional cerebral blood flow in focal cortical epilepsy. Archs Neurol. *33:* 527–535 (1976).
7 Ingvarm D.H.: Regional cerebral blood flow in focal cortical epilepsy. Stroke *4:* 359–360 (1973).
8 Ingvar, D.H.: Abnormal distribution of cerebral activity in chronic schizophrenia. A neurophysiological interpretation; in Baxter, Melnechuk, Perspectives in schizophrenia research (Raven Press, New York 1980).
9 Ingvar, D.H.; Brun, A.; Hagberg, B.; Gustafson, L.: Regional cerebral blood flow in the dominant hemisphere in confirmed cases of Alzheimer's disease, Pick's disease and multi-infarct dementia. Relationships to clinical symptomatology and neuropathological findings; in Katzman, Terry, Bick, Alzheimer's disease. Senile dementia and related disorders, pp. 203–211 (Raven Press, New York 1978).
10 Ingvar, D.H.; Franzén, G.: Cerebral activity in chronic schizophrenia. Lancet *ii* (1974).
11 Ingvar, D.H.; Franzén, G.: Abnormalities of regional cerebral blood flow in patients with mental deterioration due to chronic schizophrenia. Acta psychiat. scand. *50:* 425–462 (1974).
12 Ingvar, D.H.; Gadea-Ciria, M.: Assessment of severe damage to the brain by multi-regional measurements of cerebral blood flow; in Outcome of severe damage to the central nervous system. A Ciba Symposium (Elsevier, Amsterdam 1975).
13 Ingvar, D.H.; Lübbers, D.W.; Siesjö, B.: Measurement of oxygen tension on the surface of the cerebral cortex of the cat during hyperoxia and hypoxia. Acta physiol. scand. *48:* 373–381 (1960).
14 Jackson, J.H.: On epilepsy and epileptiform convulsions; in Taylor, Selected writings of John Hughlings Jackson, vol. 1 (Hodder & Stoughton, London 1931).
15 Kuhl, D.; Engel, J.; Phelps, M.; Selin, C.: Patterns of local cerebral metabolism and perfusion in partial epilepsy by emission computed tomography of 18-F-fluorodeoxyglucose and 13-N-ammonia; in Gotoh, Nagai, Tazaki, Cerebral blood flow and metabolism, pp. 538–539 (Munksgaard, Copenhagen 1979).
16 Lassen, N.A.; Feinberg, I.; Lane, M.H.: Bilateral studies of cerebral oxygen uptake in young and aged normal subjects and in patients with organic dementia. J. clin. Invest. *39:* 491–500 (1960).
17 Reivich, M.; Kuhl, D.; Wolf, A.; Greenberg, J.; Phelps, M.; Ido, T.; Casella, V.; Fowler, J.; Hoffman, E.; Alavi, A.; Som, P.; Sokoloff, L.: The 18-F-fluorodeoxyglucose method for the measurement of local cerebral glucose utilization in man. Circulation Res. *44:* 127–137 (1979).

David H. Ingvar, MD, Department of Clinical Neurophysiology, University Hospital,
S–221 85 Lund (Sweden)

Instructions to Authors

General observations: Only original papers written in English should be sent to:
Prof. Dr. *H.E. Kaeser*, Neurologische Universitätsklinik, Kantonsspital Basel, Petersgraben 4, CH–4031 Basel (Switzerland).
All manuscripts are subject to editorial review. They should be submitted in quadruplicate (with four sets of illustrations of which one is an original), typewritten on one side of the paper only and double-spaced with a wide margin. Manuscripts are received with the explicit understanding that they are not under simultaneous consideration by any other publication. It is the author's responsibility to obtain permission to reproduce illustrations, tables, etc. from other publications. Accepted papers become the permanent property of 'European Neurology' and may not be reproduced by any means, in whole or in part without the written consent of both the author and the publisher.

Arrangement:

Title page: The first page of each paper should carry the title (main title underlined), the authors' names and the name of the institute where the work was done. A short title for use as running head is also to be provided.

Key words: For indexing purposes, a list of 3–10 key words in English must be given.

Abstract: Each paper must have an abstract of up to 10 lines.

Small type: Paragraphs which can or must be set in smaller type (case histories, test methods, etc.) should be indicated with a 'p' (petit) in the margin on the left-hand side.

Footnotes: They should be avoided. If essential, they appear at the bottom of the respective page and must be numbered consecutively.

Tables and illustrations: Tables (numbered in Roman numerals) and illustrations (numbered in Arabic numerals) should be prepared on separate sheets. They must have a heading resp. a legend, also prepared on separate sheets. For the preparation of blocks, good drawings and original photographs should be submitted; negatives or xerox copies cannot be used. If possible, several illustrations should be grouped on one block for reproduction (max. size 140 × 190 mm) or crop marks should be given. On the back of each illustration, it's number, the author's name as well as 'top' and 'bottom' must be indicated. Colored illustrations are reproduced at the authors' expense.

References: The list of references should include only those publications which are cited in the text. They must be arranged alphabetically (citation by name and year) or numbered consecutively (citation by number).
a) Papers published in periodicals: 1. All authors' surnames ('et al.' is not sufficient) with initials of first names; 2. Full title of paper; 3. Journal abbreviation; 4. Volume (in Arabic numerals, underlined and followed by a colon); 5. First and last page; 6. Year of publication in brackets. Example: McIntosh, J.; Hansen, P.; Ziegler, J.; Penny, R.: Defective immune and phagocytic functions in uraemia and renal transplantation. Int. Archs Allergy appl. Immun. 51: 529–540 (1976).
b) Books: 1. Authors' surnames with initials of first names; 2. Full title; 3. In brackets, name and domicile of publishers and year of publication. Example: Pollack, R.S.: Tumor surgery of the head and neck (Karger, Basel 1975).

Full address: The exact postal address complete with postal code of the senior author must be given. Should correspondence be handled by someone other, it should be indicated accordingly.

Further details: Authors may consult our leaflet 'Rules for the Preparation of Manuscripts'. This may be obtained free of charge from the Publishers S. Karger AG, P.O. Box, CH–4009 Basel (Switzerland).

Page charges: There is no page charge for papers of 5 printed pages or less. Additional pages or fraction thereof are charged to the authors at SFr. 175.– / US $ 105.00 / DM 194.– per page. The alloted size of a paper is equal to approx. 10 manuscript pages (including tables, illustrations and references).

Galley proofs: They will be sent to the first-named author unless otherwise indicated and should be returned with the least possible delay. Alterations made in galley proofs, other than the corrections of printers' errors, will be charged to the author. No page proofs will be supplied.

Reprints: They are available against payment. Order forms with a price list will be sent with the galley proofs. Orders submitted after the issue is printed are subject to considerably higher prices. Allow four weeks from date of publication for delivery of reprints (surface mail; airmail delivery on request and at charge).

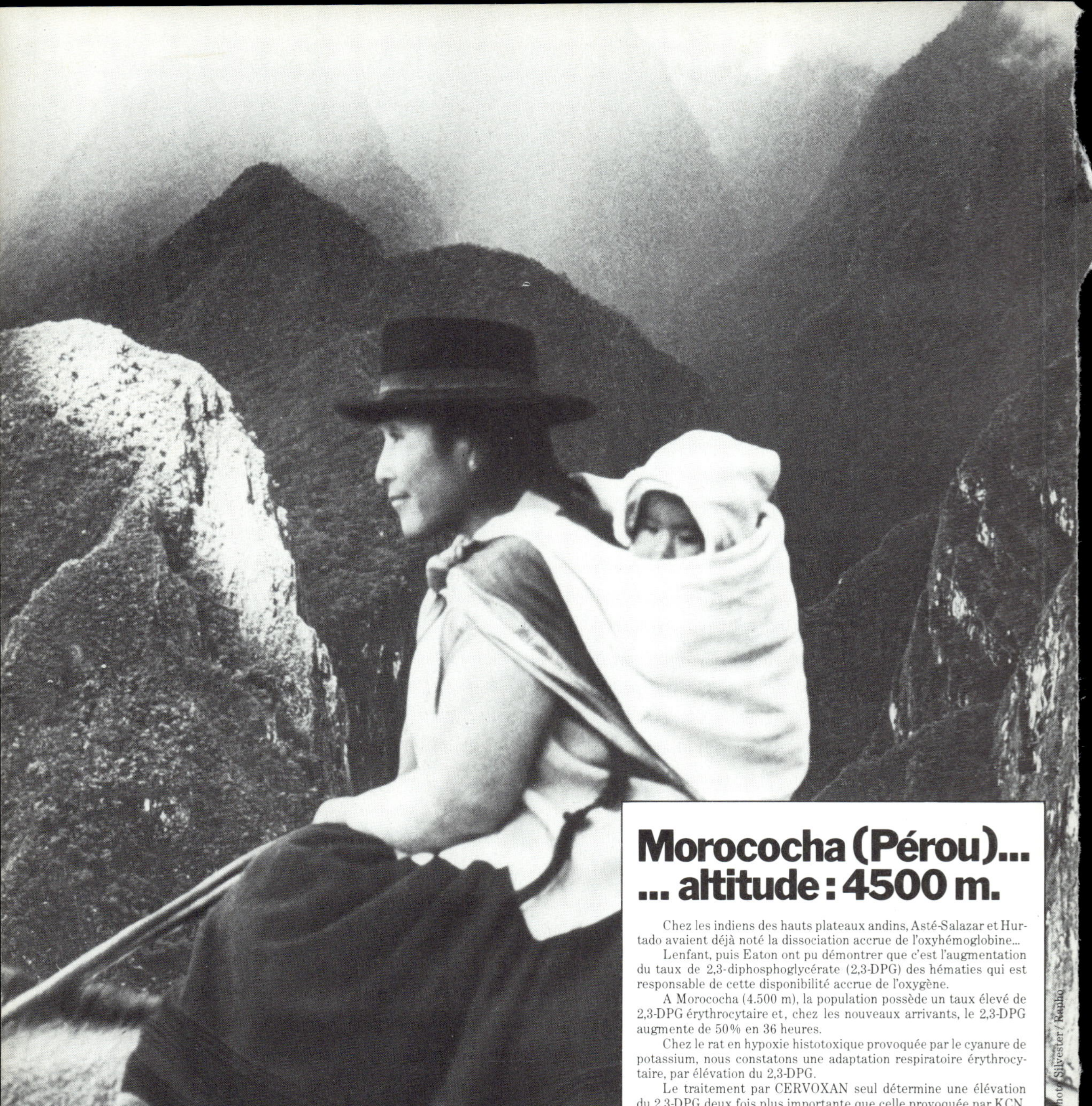

PROPRIÉTÉS : La 1-éburnamonine augmente le Pouvoir Oxyphorique Sanguin, c'est-à-dire la capacité du sang à délivrer l'oxygène aux tissus. • Au niveau pulmonaire : elle augmente la fixation de l'oxygène (PO_2 artérielle) • Au niveau érythrocytaire : elle favorise la possibilité de déformation des hématies (augmentation de l'ATP), elle augmente la dissociation de l'oxyhémoglobine, donc le relargage de l'oxygène (augmentation du 2,3 - DPG). La 1-éburnamonine protège le cerveau contre les agressions hypoxiques. Elle s'oppose aux agressions cérébrales provoquées par des hypoxies de différentes natures. Elle augmente l'apport, l'extraction et la consommation cérébrale en oxygène, en glucose, ainsi que la PO_2 tissulaire corticale. INDICATIONS : Troubles fonctionnels liés au vieillissement cérébral. Séquelles des accidents vasculaires ischémiques. En ophtalmologie : troubles rétiniens d'origine vasculaire. En O.R.L. : troubles cochléo-vestibulaires d'origine ischémique. CONTRE-INDICATIONS : femme enceinte ou susceptible de l'être ; néoformations cérébrales avec hypertension intra-crânienne. POSOLOGIE : traitement d'attaque les 20 premiers jours : 2 gélules le matin et 2 gélules le soir ou 1 ampoule I.M. le matin et 1 ampoule I.M. le soir. Traitement d'entretien, 3 gélules par jour. PRÉCAUTION D'EMPLOI : comme tous les médicaments de cette classe thérapeutique, CERVOXAN ne peut dispenser du traitement spécifique de l'hypertension artérielle. COÛT DU TRAITEMENT JOURNALIER : gélules : 4,66 F à 6,21 F. Injectable : 4,53 F. PRÉSENTATION - PRIX : boîte de 40 gélules contenant 20 mg de 1-éburnamonine : **62,10 F** + SHPC - A.M.M. 3202394 - boîte de 6 ampoules injectables contenant 15 mg de 1-éburnamonine : **13,60 F** + SHPC - A.M.M. 3202402 - Tableau C - Remb. S.S. à 70 %.

Laboratoires SOBIO - 15-25, boulevard de l'Amiral-Bruix
75782 Paris Cedex 16 - Tél. : 502.12.20

F 81083